I0830205

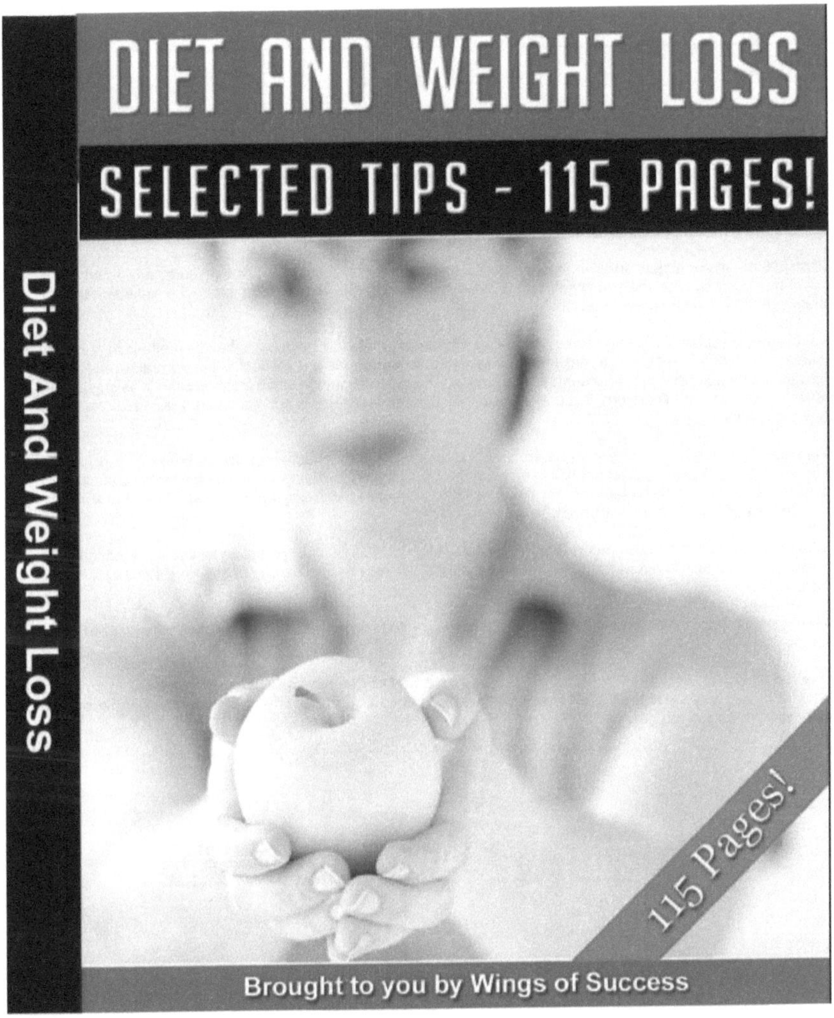

DIET AND WEIGHT LOSS

SELECTED TIPS - 115 PAGES!

Diet And Weight Loss

115 Pages!

Brought to you by Wings of Success

DISCLAIMER AND TERMS OF USE AGREEMENT:

(Please Read This Before Using This Report)

This information is not presented by a medical practitioner and is for educational and informational purposes only. The content is not intended to be a substitute for professional medical advice, diagnosis, or treatment. Always seek the advice of your physician or other qualified health provider with any questions you may have regarding a medical condition. Never disregard professional medical advice or delay in seeking it because of something you have read.

Since natural and/or dietary supplements are not FDA approved, they must be accompanied by a two-part disclaimer on the product label: that the statement has not been evaluated by FDA and that the product is not intended to "diagnose, treat, cure or prevent any disease.

The author and publisher of this course and the accompanying materials have used their best efforts in preparing this course. The author and publisher make no representation or warranties with respect to the accuracy, applicability, fitness, or completeness of the contents of this course. The information contained in this course is strictly for educational purposes. Therefore, if you wish to apply ideas contained in this course, you are taking full responsibility for your actions.

The author and publisher disclaim any warranties (express or implied), merchantability, or fitness for any particular purpose. The author and publisher shall in no event be held liable to any party for any direct, indirect, punitive, special, incidental or other consequential damages arising directly or indirectly from any use of this material, which is provided "as is", and without warranties.

As always, the advice of a competent legal, tax, accounting, medical or other professional should be sought. The author and publisher do not warrant the performance, effectiveness or applicability of any sites listed or linked to in this course.

All links are for information purposes only and are not warranted for content, accuracy or any other implied or explicit purpose.

This report is © Copyrighted by Wings Of Success. No part of this may be copied, or changed in any format, or used in any way other than what is outlined within this course under any circumstances. Violators would be prosecuted severely.

<u>Click Here To Visit Our Website</u>

SPECIAL SECRET RESOURCE!

Weight Loss For Teens - Secrets To Effective Teen Weight Management Revealed

Do You Shy Away From Handsome Guys Who Flaunt Fat-free Muscular Bodies? Do You Find It Embarrassing To Shed Your Clothes At The Swimming Pool? Frustrated With The Way You Look In The Mirror? Fret Not!

Finally Revealed! Some Little-known But Highly Effective Tips To Shed Those Ugly Pounds! Achieve Your Dream Shape, Look Sexy, And Flaunt Your Body Like Any Other Model! Your Friends Will Wonder If You Are Really The One They Knew... !

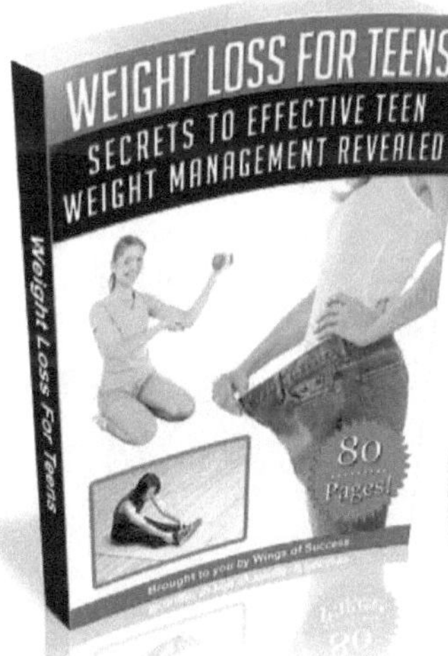

AVAILABLE ONLY FOR A VERY LIMITED TIME!

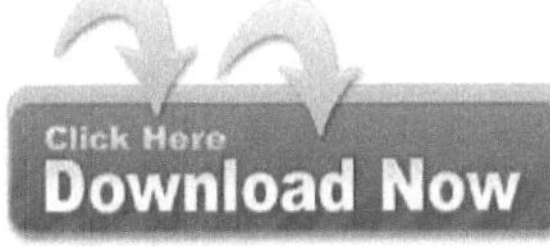

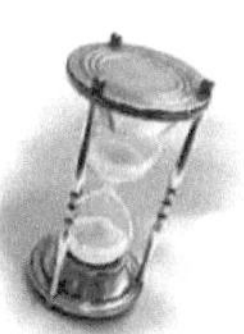

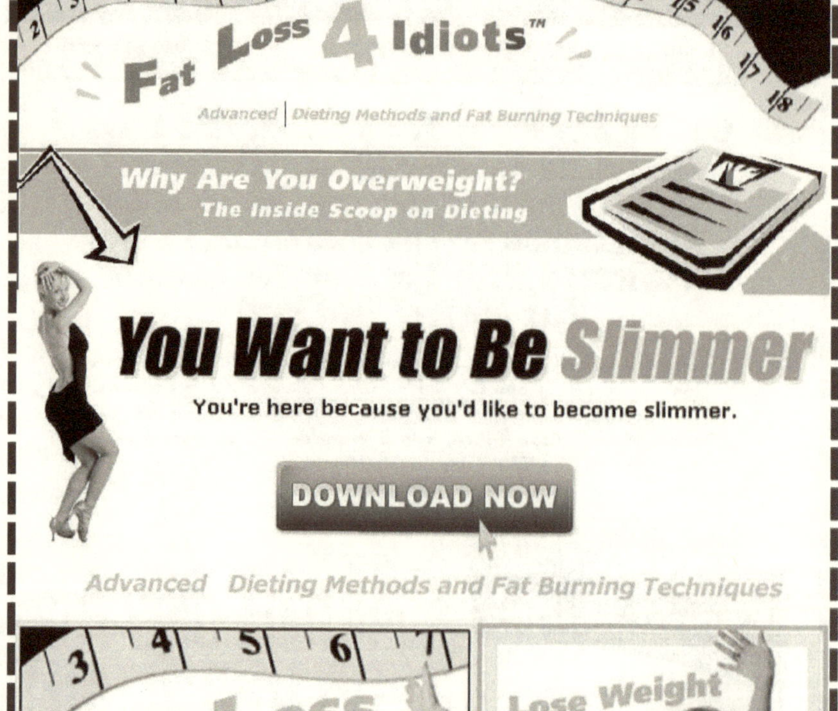
Fat Loss 4 Idiots™
Advanced | Dieting Methods and Fat Burning Techniques
Why Are You Overweight?
The Inside Scoop on Dieting
You Want to Be Slimmer
You're here because you'd like to become slimmer.
DOWNLOAD NOW
Advanced   Dieting Methods and Fat Burning Techniques
Fat Loss 4 Idiots
Lose 9 lbs. in 11 Days
Lose Weight
Get Slim

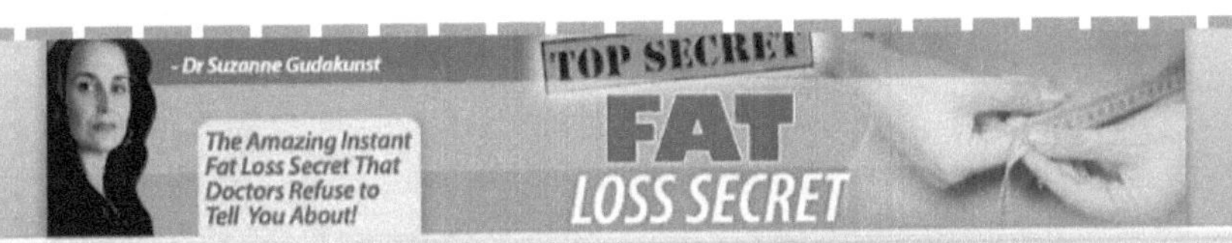

World-Famous TV Lady Doctor comes forth and blows the lid off the conspiracy to keep you unhealthy, fat & just plain sick...

Shocking Proof!

Here's the real reason you're fat...

"The Reason You Can't Lose Weight has Nothing to Do With Your *Will-Power, Over-Eating* or the *Right Diet!* ... The Reason You are Fat and Unhealthy Is Because You Have Disgusting *Plaque* and Horrible Little *'CRITTERS'* Living in Your Guts!"

"...And Now I'm Going to Show You How to Get Rid of All of It so You Can Shed 10 lbs, 25 lbs, 50 lbs even 100 lbs or more - and Keep It Off FOREVER!!"

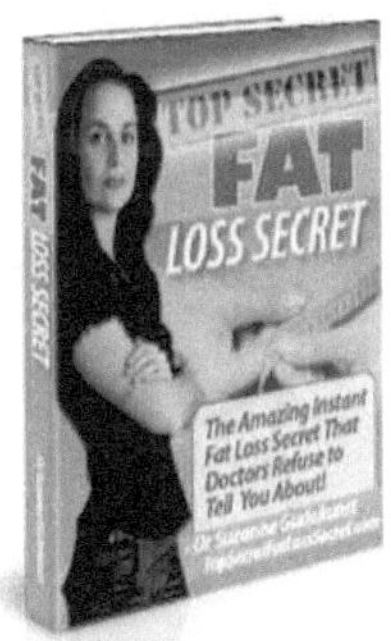

TOP SECRET
....
Fat Loss Secret

DOWNLOAD NOW

Contents

Some Tips To Lose 10 Pounds

Although some people find themselves dealing with more serious weight problems, most people who want to lose a little weight are relatively healthy. If you want to lose 10 pounds, there's a good chance that those pounds were gained very slowly of the course of many months - the weight doesn't represent a problem as much as a few times during the past year where you overindulged (usually the holidays) and failed to make up for it. Here are some tips to lose those 10 pounds:

Pick Your Time

Weight loss involves very personal issues for most people, and is closely related to their self esteem. It is crucial that you attempt to lose 10 pounds at the appropriate time - at a time where you otherwise feel good and satisfied with your life. If you try and lose 10 pounds during a period of time in your life where you have a lot of stress or other distracting things going on, you drastically increase your chances of failure, which will only make things worse.

Change Your Diet

Try as much as possible to balance your diet. This doesn't mean that you have to starve yourself -- rather make a point of getting no more the 30% of your calories from fat. Eat more fruits and vegetables and try to add as much variety to your diet as possible. Try new things, and new meal ideas.

Keep Track Of Your Progress

The problem with dieting for many people, especially in the early stages, is that even if the diet is working they can't see any results. It's hard to really notice if you lose 1 pound. For this reason it's important that your track your progress, so you can have a good sense of the accomplishments you've made. By calculating how many calories you've eaten and how much you've burned through exercise each and every day, you can track how many calories (and ultimately how much weight) you are losing.

Do It With Friends

A great and fun way to help you stick with your plan is to undertake your project of losing 10 pounds with a friend. Not only will you be able to provide support for each other and track each other's progress, but you'll be able to engage in fun exercise activities together.

Make Your Plan Realistic

It's important that you set achievable goals for yourself. For example, with just some basic changes in your lifestyle and eating habits, you can lose 1 pound a week. There's no need to be in a huge rush to lose weight, and trying to lose weight quickly often requires a regimen that is difficult to keep up. For most people, it is healthier to lose weight slowly than with drastic dietary changes.

Many people would like to lose 10 pounds, and almost anyone can if they follow the advice above. By avoiding a "quick fix" and sticking with long term healthy choices, you'll find your project to lose 10 pounds will leave you not only thinner, but healthier and feeling better about yourself.

Diet

We've probably all found ourselves, at one time or another in our lives, wanting to lose some weight. Whether you're trying to take off some pounds gained during the holiday season, preparing for a summer trip, or simply looking for a way to feel more fit and healthy, trying to lose weight is rarely a bad idea.

This is the most obvious starting point, yet one that is commonly overlooked. Most people, when they're trying to lose 10 pounds, think of things like cutting out junk food and avoiding snacks. While this is no doubt important, it is not necessary to starve yourself if you're looking to lose 10 pounds.

The most important things to consider in terms of your diet are balance and proportion. If you want to lose 10 pounds for good, you're going to have to think in terms of your overall eating habits. By changing your eating habits permanently for the better, the weight you lose will stay lost.

Your daily intake of food should include a well balanced proportion of protein, carbohydrates, and vegetables. Variety is the key to this. Ask yourself: can you name more than 3 vegetables that you eat regularly and enjoy? Or more generally: how many different "meals" do you make for yourself during an average week? Most people in answering these questions will realize that there's not as much variety to their diet as they may of thought.

When trying to lose 10 pounds, you also have to try to be in tune with your body as much as possible. You probably don't realize, unless you think about it, how little you adhere to your body's needs. Most people eat roughly the same amount at the same time every day. While this is convenient, it doesn't necessarily sync up with what you need. Ask yourself: are you always hungry when you eat? Do you stop eating when you're full, or do you eat all of whatever you've made?

These simple changes in dietary habits can work wonders, and render you goal of losing 10 pounds less daunting than it probably seems.

A Diet To Lose 10 Pounds

Almost all of us at one time or another have wanted to lose weight. Some people are motivated by the arrival of summer, while others have set new year's resolutions or are trying to work off some holiday weight. Whatever the reasons, the desire to lose 10 pounds is a common one, and can be achieved through dietary habits.

When looking to lose 10 pounds, it's important to understand that your dietary habits are just that: habits. In other words, there's probably not only a lot of things that you eat that you don't give much thought to, but also a lot of ways that you east that you don't think about. By changing your dietary habits you will not only lose weight, but you will be able to keep that weight off.

Before you look at specific diets to lose 10 pounds, think about your eating routines. It's important to eat a wide variety of foods, and to eat in proportion. A sure sign that you need to incorporate more variety and balance into your diet is if you can only think of a few "standard meals" that you cook for yourself, or if you can only name a few vegetables that you like. Not only will adding more variety to your diet help you lose those ten pounds, it will provide you with an opportunity to expand the range of meals you can cook.

The other thing to consider when trying to lose ten pounds is your eating habits themselves. We all naturally fall into routines, and there's a good chance that you eat roughly the same amount of food at the same time every day. While this is convenient, it's not necessarily what your body desires. When you eat, make a point of eating slowly and of stopping when you're full. As simple as it sounds, many people eat what they prepare, when they prepare it, regardless of whether or not they are hungry. By learning to understand how your body is relating to the food you put in it, you'll be able to make permanent dietary choices that result in weight loss without being very restrictive.

Now, in some cases you're going to want to lose 10 pounds fairly quickly. If you find yourself in this position consider the following small dietary changes:

- ***Stop eating cream cheese:*** while you probably already know that cream cheese isn't healthy, you might not know that a toasted bagel can taste great without it.

- Remove Chicken Skin: A simple way to reduce fat is to get in the habit of removing the skin from chicken breasts. You'll find this easy to do by scraping a sharp knife perpendicularly across the surface of the breast.

- Skip Salted Peanuts: Peanuts are a great and filling snack when you're hungry, but try switching to the salt-free variety. You'll be surprised how quickly you get used to them - in fact you'll soon find salted peanuts unappetizing.

These are just some of the small changes you can make to your diet in order to lose 10 pounds. But Remember: if you want to keep the weight off, you'll have to make some of the more permanent dietary changes listed earlier as well.

Lose 10 Pounds By Adjusting Your Eating Habits

Whether you're trying to lose some holiday weight, made a new year's resolution, or simply want to look and feel healthier, a weight loss attempt is rarely a bad idea. A good place to start for most people is to set a goal to lose 10 pounds. To lose 10 pounds should be easily attainable for most people, and often with less work than you think.

When people think about losing weight, the first thing that usually comes to mind is diet. Your diet is, of course, one of the most primary influences on your overall weight, and you would be ill-advised to overlook it in your attempt to lose 10 pounds. Rather then thinking only about your diet, however, you should think about your eating habits as a whole. By looking at the bigger picture you will be able to effect more permanent changes on your weight.

It some cases, and for some people, it is possible to lose 10 pounds quickly through some hard and fast dietary rules. The problem, though, is that these rules are likely going to be restrictive, so there's a good chance that they're going to be hard to stick to. Not only that, but if you do stray from the restrictions, those 10 pounds are going to come back quickly.

A much better way to try and lose 10 pounds is to adjust your overall eating habits. While it may ultimately take a little longer to lose the weight this way, the weight loss is far more likely to be permanent. To lose 10 pounds by adjusting your eating habits, you have to first give those habits close scrutiny. If you stop and think about it, you'll probably be surprised how often you eat when you are not actually hungry. For example, many people eat in front of the TV not because they are hungry, but out of habit. In the same manner, you probably eat the same amount of food at the same times every day, with little regard for your hunger.

The way you're going to lose 10 pounds, then, is to listen more closely to your body. The stomach sends very clear signals, but they are slow: it is a rule of thumb that you don't "feel" full until 20 minutes after you actually are full. This is why people get overstuffed: we've all had the experience of wanting one more helping, only to regret it 20 minutes later.

So you should make an attempt to eat your food more slowly and to savor it - this will allow your body more time to signal to you how full it is. Also make sure to stop eating when you're full - you can always save leftovers - because there's no reason to eat food simply because it's there.

Altering your eating habits is one of the most effective and easiest ways that you can lose 10 pounds. For many people, weight loss will occur simply be reducing your intake of food. This doesn't mean you have to starve yourself, it just means not eating when you're not hungry. Following the guidelines above will allow you to permanently change your eating habits, and more importantly: to lose 10 pounds, and keep it off.

Exercise

This is another fundamental step in losing weight. You're not going to be able to easily lose 10 pounds though dietary habits alone. Exercise must become a part of your lifestyle.

The problem many people face is that they feel they don't have the time for exercise. Granted, not everyone may have time to get to the gym every day, but there are many things you can do at home: besides sit-ups and other equipment-free exercise, equipment like a treadmill, Stairmaster, or exercise-bike can allow you to lose weight without a gym membership.

In terms of the time involved in trying to lose 10 pounds, many of you may be saying that you barely have enough time in the day as it is, let alone adding exercise to the mix. If you have an exercise-bike, treadmill, or other similar equipment however, your exercise routine can easily be combined with other activities you enjoy and make time for, like watching television or listening to music. In this way you'll find exercising doesn't require that you make time as much is it requires you change your way of doing activities you already do.

Exercise Is The Best Way To Lose Weight

Even though thousands of overweight teenagers seem to have gained their weight overnight, it is the result of a lifestyle without exercise. As a result, it is impossible to see immediate results from starting a habit of good physical fitness.

In the current age of information and technology, all the diets and man-made methods of weightless do not come close to good, old fashioned physical activity.

Unlike diets and pill popping, exercise causes a dramatic increase in your metabolism, which comes from your increase in endurance, allowing for a long term solution for weight loss.

Diets and pills can cause certain side effects, where as the only possible side effect that can come from exercise is muscle strain, and that can be avoided through proper stretching before and after a workout.

With the economy rising and falling, paying a ton of money on diets and pills are unnecessary due to the extremely cost affective method of weight loss found in exercising. The reason for this is due to the physical activity needed can be done at the comfort of your home, such as jogging, push ups, sit ups, and other such exercises.

If you do not know any exercises or strategies to help with your weight loss, you can spend a fraction of the cost for diets and pills on a Gym membership where they provide programs and personal trainers to assist you reaching your physical goals.

For example, gearing up for your daily activity can be done by jogging a few miles on a treadmill or utilizing the variety of other available machines.

If having a trainer is too awkward or just too expensive for you, take only the first few lessons and gleam all the needed information from the provided trainer so you can learn how to exercise on your own. Most Gyms also offer fitness classes free with membership, which prove to be more than helpful, educating you in the methods of Tae Bo, Pilates, yoga and Aerobics.

Since shyness is common among teenagers, there are hundreds of fitness videos available online. These are always helpful, as it only holds a one time purchasing cost and all you need to do establish a time of physical activity at home. Remember to drink lots of water while working out at home. Most Gyms supply water sources right in the facility, however while in the comfort of home it is easy to forget to keep hydrated. If you forget, heatstroke or dehydration is common side effects.

There is no shame in easing your way into a physically active life style. Sometimes it is Doctor recommended, due to the body's needs not matching your will to jump right into the workout. Since this is the case, get a check up with your personal physician and get their analyses on your physical condition and go from there.

One of the great methods to keep up this new found lifestyle of fitness is to engage in sports. Do not hide from the court anymore... dive in and race up and down the gym. This speeds up your heart rate and adds to your endurance levels, not to mention the loss in calories.

These are some practical methods on how teens can lose weight. Remember, everyone has the potential to live healthy; we just need a small shove in the right direction.

Lose 10 Pounds By Jogging

For the vast majority of people, weight gain is a very slow, almost imperceptible process. Most of us are familiar with the experience of stepping on a scale and wondering just where, exactly, did those pounds come from. For most people, the weight comes from times in the past year where they indulged. What happens is that you indulge for a week or two (vacation, Christmas) and then go back to your normal lifestyle -- you do nothing to lose the weight. So these small weight gains stay with you and build up over time. For this reason almost anyone would love to lose 10 pounds at some point, and a great way to do so is by jogging.

Depending on who you talk to, jogging is considered the best exercise to lose weight. The reason is because the high intensity of jogging burns a lot of calories. If you're looking to lose 10 pounds, there are a lot worse things you could try than a half-hour jog a few times a week.

Jogging is also preferable for many people because it incorporates exercise in a more interesting way: trying to lose 10 pounds by going to the gym 3 times a week isn't a whole lot of fun. It will certainly feel like "work" as you count off the minutes of your workout. Jogging, on the other hand, requires nothing but a pair of shoes, and allows you to enjoy some scenery.

One of the problems people face when trying to lose 10 pounds is incorporating exercise into their daily routines. Most of us are busy enough as it is, and can't find the time to go to the gym at scheduled intervals. If you're trying to lose 10 pounds, you'll find that jogging is a much more flexible activity - you don't have to drive to the gym: you can do it wherever and whenever you want.

While jogging is an excellent way to lose 10 pounds and increase your fitness level, you should keep in mind that it is harder on the body then a lot of other physical activities. Jogging involves lurching your full weight around repeatedly - this is precisely why it's such a good workout - and this can cause stress on the joints in your knees and feet. You should also keep in mind that jogging is an intense physical activity, so if you're starting from a very low level of fitness it may be a little too much, and you may want to work up to it.

As long as you keep the above in mind though, you'll find jogging an excellent way to lose 10 pounds. As an added bonus, jogging is recognized as one of the best ways to maintain weight as well, so you don't have to worry about a diet that gains all the weight back once it's stopped. And even though you may be jogging primarily to lose those 10 pounds, you'll also be doing wonders for the health of your heart and cardiovascular system.

Lose 10 Pounds By Biking

So you want to lose weight. All of us do at some point and losing weight is a great way to both look and feel better. Not only that, but you'll feel better about yourself and have more confidence. A great goal to set for yourself when initially trying to lose weight is to try and lose 10 pounds. This should be an attainable goal for almost anyone.

So where do you start? Most people, when they think of weight loss, think of unappetizing diets or strenuous exercise regimens, but it doesn't have to be that way. If you're looking to lose 10 pounds while still having fun and getting some fresh air, look instead to what was probably one of your favorite childhood activities: bicycling.

There are many benefits to biking, but the main one is that it's really the only form of exercise that can also function as transportation. The reason it's difficult for many people to lose weight is because to try work too much time into their already busy lifestyles. For example, let's say your plan is to lose 10 pounds by getting a gym membership and going a few times a week. While this may be great at first, there's a good chance that it's going to start interfering with other commitments: one day you have to stay late at work so you skip gym; one day you have to pick up your son from soccer practice so you skip. Eventually it becomes easy to break the gym routine, because it's always going to seem like some "extra" that you don't always have time for.

Now say instead of going to the gym to lose those 10 pounds you decide to bike to work. While it may take a little longer to lose the weight, by biking to work you're really losing no time at all. If you live in a city there's a good chance that it's not going to take you a whole lot longer than a car trip does. So basically you get to lose 10 pounds "for free", as it were, because you don't have to make time for exercise.

When you engage in most other forms of exercise, you're engaging in it exclusively: you're not getting anything else done when you're at the gym. With biking, on the other hand, the exercise is almost a secondary bonus to the primary function of getting somewhere you need to go. Add to this the fact that you're saving money on transportation and doing good for the environment, it's hard to argue against biking as one of the best forms of exercise.

By simply biking to and from work every day you should be able to lose 10 pounds fairly quickly without affecting your schedule too much. If your employer is a far enough distance away from you that you must drive, consider instead using a bike for errands outside of work. And if you want to really lose those 10 pounds quickly, start biking for recreation too - some weekend bike riding will do wonders for weight loss.

How To Lose 10 Pounds By Exercising

Almost all of us at some point in our lives are going to want to lose some weight. Not only will losing weight make you feel and look better, it will make you feel better about yourself and help your self-confidence. A good starting point for most people is to try and lose 10 pounds, and for many people this can be easily achieved through exercise.

Before beginning your attempt to lose 10 pounds, sit down and take a look at your lifestyle. Are you active? Do you watch a lot of TV? Do you spend your day in an office in front of a computer? Most people don't get nearly the amount of exercise they should be getting, and although this is a bad thing, it also means that your body will respond quickly to an increase in exercise.

The reason exercise seems difficult to most people is that it can seem like more work than it actually is. A lot of people who want to lose 10 pounds by exercising immediately think of a gym, and a regimen that they don't have time for. While there is no doubt that going a gym is one of the best ways you can exercise, it is far from the only one.

Most of us live very inactive lives. Think about it: you probably drive to work, sit for 8 hours, and drive home. Once you get home you're tired enough that you simply want to "relax." It may seem difficult to work exercise into this routine, but you'll find it's not that hard at all. By simply acquiring an exercise bike, Stairmaster, or the like, you can watch TV or listen to music while you're excising. This is a great way to "wind-down" after a day of work - plus if you're going to be watching TV anyway, you're not losing any time, you're simply doing two things at once.

Another good idea is to try and get some exercise while you're at work. Think how often you end up staying in your office on your lunch break. Instead, why not take a walk? It may not seem like much, but if you did that every day, you'd be walking 5 hours a week, which is a pretty great start towards getting some more exercise. On the weekends and in the evenings, take up a sport or an active hobby like hiking. The key is to find ways that you can get exercise while also doing things you enjoy.

You can lose 10 pounds fairly quickly by starting a serious exercise regimen, of course, but that's not necessarily the best way to do it. If you make your exercise like work, it'll start to feel like work, and it will become tempting to put it off and avoid it. If you incorporate exercise into your daily routine, however, it won't seem like work at all - it will be fun. And the best part of all is that the more you exercise the more energy you'll have: instead of being tired when you come home from work, you'll feel like doing something active. Before you know it those 10 pounds you lost might become 20.

Lifestyle

Now you not only want to lose 10 pounds, you want those 10 pounds to stay lost, right? A way to ensure success with keeping that weight off is to make some lifestyle changes.

Everyone becomes accustomed to their routines, and it's difficult to force changes on those routines. One of the reasons many people fail with a task like losing 10 pounds is that it seems to require too much discipline and work. While a certain amount of stick-to-itiveness is no doubt necessary, you'll find it much easier to lose weight if you incorporate changes into your lifestyle. A diet and exercise routine is almost certain to fail if it conflicts with your daily routines.

For example, if you live a reasonable distance from work, try biking instead of driving. What you're doing here is incorporating exercise in to your normal routine: work is something you go to every day anyway --all you're doing is changing the way you get there. Changing the way you do something that you already do is far more convenient than starting something new, and biking to work is much easier to incorporate into your lifestyle then going to the gym every day.

The same principle can be applied to your eating habits. Do you pack a lunch for work or eat out? If you eat out, chances are you're going to be eating something less healthy than you would make for yourself, and probably a larger portion as well. By getting up a little earlier each morning and preparing your own lunch, you're not only saving money, but your incorporating a healthy eating choice in your routine. This is much easier to do then having a list in your head and constantly reminding yourself of what you can and can't eat.

Not only are lifestyle changes easier to enforce than hard and fast diet rules, they're also more permanent. Simply look at your daily routine for places where you could incorporate a bit of exercise: take the stairs instead of the elevator; walk instead of taking the bus. These changes will not only make you lose weight, but you'll feel healthier and better without having to constantly chastise yourself for breaking dieting "rules."

Making Lifestyle Changes To Lose 10 Pounds

So you want to lose some weight. Almost all of us have felt this way at some time or another. Maybe it's some holiday weight you want to work off, or maybe you've just decided that you would feel and look better with a little less bulk. Whatever the reason, losing weight can sometimes be difficult. It's often the case that you find yourself dealing with a very restrictive diet that is difficult to stick to, or other inconveniences. You can avoid much of this, however, by making some lifestyle changes that incorporate more healthy activities into your daily routine.

Although everyone will likely be tempted to try and lose their 10 pounds as quickly as possible, unless you feel for some reason that this is absolutely necessary, it's better to take a long term approach. If you want to lose 10 pounds quickly, it's likely that you're going to have to make a restrictive and drastic diet change that will be hard to implement. This also means there's a good chance you will simply put the weight back on when you diet is over, or when you (inevitably) lapse from it.

A far better long term solution is making some lifestyle changes. Not only will this be an easier way to lose 10 pounds, but those 10 pounds will stay lost. The reason that lifestyle changes are an effective way to lose weight is that you don't have to alter your daily routine too much. Many people find the exercise regimens and diet changes involved in quick weight loss unrealistic - you never have enough hours in the day as it is, so it's hard to make more for exercise.

The best place to start In your attempt to lose 10 pounds is to look at things you do every day. First and foremost for most people is going to work. Many people live close enough to their employers to bike, but choose instead to drive. By biking to work you will not only be getting exercise and working towards your goal of losing 10 pounds, you will be saving money and doing a good thing for the environment. Try and think of other small changes in a similar vein: take the stairs instead of the elevator, go for a walk on your lunch break instead of sitting at your desk. Although these chances may seem small and suspiciously convenient, they will go along way towards losing weight.

The other more pro-active way to lose 10 pounds through a lifestyle change is to engage in more athletic activities. Take up a sport, or go hiking on weekends. The beauty of this is that these things are entirely recreational: you're having fun at the same time that you're losing weight. It's much easier and more enjoyable to commit to going on a hike every weekend or playing tennis with a friend than it is to sit alone in gym: after all, there's a reason they call it "work"ing out.

Lifestyle changes go a long way towards losing weight, and anyone who incorporates some of the changes listed above should find themselves able to lose 10 pounds.

Lose 10 Pounds By Getting Up Early

Weight gain can be a very slow process. For most people, it is a matter of one pound here, one pound there, and the next thing you know you're 10 pounds heavier. This is why almost everyone, at one point or another, will want to lose 10 pounds. To lose 10 pounds is very realistic for almost everyone, and is achievable though some small changes in diet and by exercising more. The vast majority of people, with their busy schedules, get little or no exercise, so even a small bit of regular exercise should be able to achieve noticeable results. If we don't have time to exercise a great deal, though, we're going to want to maximize the effectiveness of the exercise we do get, and a great way to do that is by exercising in the morning.

There are two main reasons why you can more easily lose 10 pounds by exercising in the morning. The first has to do with the fact that it is much easier to build into your daily routine. One of the keys to losing weight by exercise is to do it regularly, which many people find difficult: it's always hard to find time. So a great reason for exercising in the morning is that you'll have very little distraction. In many ways, you are literally "making time" for the exercise by starting your day earlier.

Now, in terms of your goal to lose 10 pounds, morning exercise will be more effective because you will be burning calories from fat already in your system. This principle is based, of course, on the idea that you don't eat before you exercise. The way you're going to lose 10 pounds is by burning fat, and when you exercise your body normally burns both fat and carbohydrates. Now it gets a little more complicated: your body's main and preferred energy source is carbohydrates, so when you exercise you will (more or less) burn carbohydrates first, and then your body will dip into its fat reserves.

Carbohydrates come from your meals, so when you exercise at a normal time of the day your body will have plenty of carbohydrates to burn. In trying to lose 10 pounds, however, you're hoping to burn fat. If you exercise in the morning on an empty stomach, you're burning energy at a time when your body's carbohydrate levels are the lowest, and therefore more fat will be burned with the same amount of exercise. There have been studies that suggest over 250% more fat is burned when you exercise in this state.

There is never any immediate way to lose 10 pounds - ultimately, losing weight requires smart dietary decisions and a well thought out routine of exercise. By exercising in the morning, however, you will be giving yourself a distinct advantage in that battle to lose 10 pounds - you will be privy to not only a physiological advantage, but also the practical one of conducting your exercise at the beginning of the day without distraction.

Planning

If you want to lose 10 pounds, it's imperative that you have a plan. The chances of you being successful are very unlikely if you collect an odd batch of advice here and there and implement it sporadically. First, think of a realistic timeframe in which you want to lose 10 pounds. When you're doing this, keep in mind how much time you're willing to devote it, and how much you're willing to affect your daily routine: it's going to take more work to lose 10 pounds in 2 weeks than it is to lose 10 pounds in a month, for example.

Although healthy weight loss requires a balanced solution, when planning, pick which aspects of weight loss you'd like to focus on more: do you want to devote more time to exercise, and have more flexibility with your diet, or vice versa? When coming up with a weight loss plan, be realistic and think about how much time and effort you're willing to commit.

Making a weight loss plan is important because it gives you goals and something to stick to. Make your plan specific: don't say "I'm going to exercise this week," say "I'm going to exercise every day for 30 minutes when I get home from work." Try to come up with goals and expectations for yourself every day, so you can benefit from a regular sense of achievement.

The basic outline of your plan should incorporate both diet and exercise. A good way to start is to research a few healthy meals and plan to make them in your first week. This is more enjoyable than simply making a list of things you can't eat: you'll learn how to cook new things, and you'll have the satisfaction of preparing an enjoyable meal. The same goes for exercise: come up with some activities for the week. These don't have to be boring, work-type, exercise activities. Think of things like playing a sport, or taking a hike.

<u>Lose 10 Pounds - Planning And Executing</u>

There are many different reasons why someone may want to lose weight, but it's a pretty safe bet that almost everybody will want to at some point in their lives. Losing weight will make you feel and look better, and will increase your self confidence. An excellent place to start for most people is to set a goal to lose 10 pounds. Like in many other aspects of life, the key to achieving your goal - to lose 10 pounds - lies in proper planning and execution.

Everybody is different. We all have different lifestyles, schedules and abilities, and it's important that this is kept in mind when approaching your project of losing 10 pounds. Before you actually begin trying to lose the weight, you must decide on a realistic plan that is right for you. The worst thing you can do is set a plan that is difficult to achieve. If, for example, you're an extremely busy working parent, don't create a plan for yourself that entails exercising 15 hours a week, as chances are you're going to fail, which will only end up making you feel worse about yourself.

Every weight loss attempt should ideally compose both dietary changes and an increase in exercise. Depending on your situation, you may want to focus on one more than the other. If, for example, you want to lose 10 pounds but don't have time for lots of exercise, you might want to focus on your diet, which after all requires more discipline than time.

When looking at your diet, do some research and come up with some healthy meal ideas that you don't normally eat. Plan to eat these new meals on a regular basis. You want to break your plan into as many small steps as possible, so that you provide yourself with many small, achievable goals. For example, you may decide to research your new meal on Monday, buy the ingredients on Tuesday, and make it on Wednesday. Not only does this split the work up - if you leave it all to one day it's far more likely you won't have the time to do it - but it creates a constant sense of accomplishment.

Now let's say your plan to lose 10 pounds is going to be mainly through exercise. Again, don't plan to "exercise 10 hours a week" because what will probably happen is you'll put it off all week and then won't have time for it. You want to plan to exercise for an hour a day, and you want to try and incorporate that exercise into other activities.

At least half the battle with trying to lose 10 pounds is one of discipline: as anyone who has been on a diet or exercise regimen will tell you, it's easy to start a diet but hard to stick with it. The worst thing you can do when trying to lose 10 pounds is to set yourself up for failure, as this is a cycle that tends to repeat itself. By creating and executing a well thought out and realistic plan, you give yourself a huge advantage in your ultimate goal of losing 10 pounds.

Sticking To Your Plan

It is crucial, of course, to keep your goal in mind - losing 10 pounds - and to realize that it's not going to happen if you don't stick to your plan. The two vital components to sticking to your plan are to make your plan specific and realistic, and to come up with a reward system.

As much as possible, have your plan include a specific thing each and every day. For example, come up with a specific meal you're going to cook, and a specific activity for every day of the week. Not only does this give you more direction, but allows for an achievable goal every day.

Once you've come up with your specific daily goals towards losing 10 pounds, think of some rewards. Keep in mind of course, that your rewards should not include unhealthy eating or activities. Tell yourself, for example, that if you meet all your goals for a given week you're going to go a movie or attend an event you've been wanting to see.

This sticking to your plan and rewarding yourself element is often overlooked in weight loss attempts, and is why many fail. The reason has to do with the cycle of self-esteem. If you've made the decision that you want to lose 10 pounds, it's likely that you don't feel as good about yourself as you could. If you fail to meet your goals and to reward yourself, this self-doubt will increase and it will be tempting to scrap the entire weight loss attempt.

Think of your goal of losing ten pounds as a project, and think of how a business approaches a project: with very specific and regular targets that are met. Your feeling of self satisfaction will grow as you continue to meet your targets, and as you begin to feel better about yourself it will become easier to set and reach loftier goals.

Stick To A Routine And Lose 10 Pounds

Eventually, almost everyone is going to be inclined to try and lose some weight. Losing weight will not only make you feel and look better, but it will increase your self esteem and confidence. A good initial target for most people is to lose 10 pounds. By creating a routine of activity and diet, most people will be able to lose 10 pounds with little trouble.

As anyone who has tried it knows, one of the hardest things about a weight loss regimen is just that: the regimen. The reasons most diets and exercise routines fail is simply because they are difficult to stick to. One of the best things you can do to avoid this pitfall is to come up with a realistic plan before you attempt to lose 10 pounds, and to incorporate that plan into your daily routine.

It's important that you do your own research to come up with a plan that works for you, but as an example let's consider the following: let's say to lose 10 pounds your plan calls for 30 minutes of exercise 5 days a week, and to cook 3 new and healthy meals a week. None of these things should be particularly cumbersome, but if you fail to plan and organize them into your routine it will be easy for them to fall by the wayside.

Let's start with the exercise. If you want to exercise 30 minutes a day, when are you going to do it? Don't just say to yourself "whenever I can squeeze it in" as that is a guarantee that it will get squeezed out. Depending on your job and family responsibilities, it's going to be best for you to either exercise before work, at work, or after work. Exercising before or after work could entail using a stationary bike while watching TV, while exercise at work could be taking a brisk walk during your lunch hour. Whatever choice you make, make sure you stick to it. In order to lose 10 pounds you have to think of this exercise as part of your daily routine, as regular as anything else you do throughout an average day. If you don't do this, the exercise will become an "extra" thing you do, and will be the first thing dropped from your agenda when you get busy.

Now let's look at the diet in this example. You're going to lose 10 pounds by making 3 new meals a week. Again, this has to be planned and part of your routine. Decide what days you're going to cook them, decide what (earlier) days you're going to plan them and shop for them. If you fail to do this you'll find that you simply don't have the time for 3 new meals a week. And the problem, of course, is that most of us really don't "have time" for anything, so unless we make the time, it's not going to happen.

To lose 10 pounds is not as difficult as many people may think, and be careful to not get completely wrapped up in the ideas of diet and exercise. While these things are the fundamental tools to losing weight, they won't work if not properly incorporated into your daily routine.

Dealing With Fast Weight Loss Programs And Surgeries For Teenagers

Being a teenager is hard, dealing all the social pressures and the pressures of new things entering into their lives, coping with their surrounding environment.

Not only do they deal with bodily changes, hormonal and chemical compositions, but also changes in their home life, social life, which, for some, is the most complex to deal with.

Teenagers go head long into a world where the stories of ostracism and bullying are far from fictional. Depending on their popularity, the social pressures the lay upon their minds are constant and unforgiving.

Due to this, the major achievement in most social settings is to be accepted by the majority, to be popular, and, sadly, in order to do that, the ostracism involves their outward appearance.

Since the consideration of their outward appearance is so common, they dive into diets in order to loss those pounds that plant them in their unpopular status. No one desires to diet, but their craving for social acceptance is greater than the pains of rejecting their favorite meal.

It is from this place of insecurity that eating disorders form and surgical solutions are explored. Both of these methods are harmful to the body and, both, the short and long term. But, because the teenagers are able to see immediate results, these have become just a few of the most popular weight loss strategies.

The role of a parent is one of great importance in this process. It is the teenager's parents that reveal to them the criteria to making good decisions, while maintaining your understanding and support of their social position. Sadly, the majority of parents seem to oppose their teenager's decision making rather than supporting them.

Due to this fact, teenagers have been labeled as rebellious and unreachable by their parents. They close off to their guardians and attempt to live their own life, dealing with their own problems, alone. By getting involved in their lives, you will be able to witness their actions, regardless if you agree or disagree with them. Be supportive and place limits on their behavior so they do not hurt themselves. Being aware of what is really going on is key.

Just because they do not go along with your recommendations, do not shun them. Support them in their decisions and help them shop for the right surgical doctor or the next dieting phase. Allow them to watch you weigh the pros and cons to each possibility and, who knows, perhaps this will assist in dissuading them.

Your teenagers can make rational decisions when given the proper information. Give them the ability to research for themselves. Show them different testimonials of success and failures, pictures of the people that went through surgery and had a minor or major mishap. Reveal every aspect, from every perspective, and assist them in thinking rationally for themselves.

Free Weight Loss Program For Teenagers

Teen Celebrities have been placed in magazines like Vogue, moving up and down their catwalks, showing off the results of their new diets. Our teenagers, still in their most influential stage of their lives, see this and desire the same outcome.

The stars speak about their new dieting discoveries, yet Lindsey Lohan, Paris Hilton, and Hillary Duff are neglecting to mention the astronomical costs of implementing their weight loss programs, of which, for them, would only be pocket change.

Believe it or not, the most effective weight loss program can be designed by you, at home, for free!

Set your goal

Everything affects everyone differently, and this includes the many dieting programs that are available. For example, a program implemented by someone who wishes to lose 30 pounds would not be an excellent program for someone needed to lose 50. Likewise, some people require more muscle tone, where other people desperately need to ease into a physically active lifestyle.

Before you can decide anything, you must determine your weight loss goal. The internet is a vast and effective information highway, and it includes something called the Mass Index, a chart that shows the healthy weight per your individual height. Consult this before designing your personal weight loss program.

A Mixture of Exercise and Dieting

Dieting is tricky, since it requires not the abandoning of any one aspect, but a balance of your entire daily intake. A healthy balance will allow your body to adjust; however, an unhealthy balance could be potentially harmful.

Exercising could also be harmful if done excessively, causing muscle strain. The balance of both a healthy diet and a well planned exercise program is necessary for your desired healthy lifestyle.

Everything in Time

Dieting only for fast results is far from practical, as it never assists in a long term transformation. You will lose weight on these crash diets, but as time goes on, your body will crash along with the diet as you will immediately require a large amount of intake due to lack of nutrients. This is why it is better in the long run to for a plan that will allow you to loss weight at a steady pace, instead of seeking fast results.

Your Level of Commitment

The pains of change must outweigh the pains of staying the same. Figure out if you hold the commitment level required to see through this new lifestyle of a balanced diet and exercise. If you can not see yourself following through with you plans, store them for another day. Only when a commitment is present will anything be accomplished.

Healthy Way For Teens To Lose Weight

When your diet has high amounts of fats and sugars, it is an inevitability that you are going to become overweight. Ironically, it is usually those that can not seem to kick their habitual addiction for this food that desire fast results from their chosen diets.

For example, the veggie diet is a common choice for immediate results. The only issue here is teenagers, when adventuring into the world of greens and yellows only eat veggies and not any meats, thinking they are the source of fat. In fact, the proteins and other nutrients found in meats, such as chicken and fish, are necessary for a healthy lifestyle.

Because of this, teenagers would then have to over load on veggies in order to compensate for their lack of nutrients needed for healthy growth.

Another method is drinking herbal tea. Even though this is a healthy thing to do in moderation, the tea acts as a natural laxative, causing you to run to the bathroom more often than usual. This may be strategic in the teenage mind for weight loss, but what really happens is the laying of groundwork for eventual colon problems.

Television ads are very convincing to the Teenager. Every once and a while a new diet pops up on the shopping network, promising a two week solution to dropping those unwanted pounds.

Since these diets usually deal with fewer calories in your diet, a teenager needs every ounce of their calorie intake due to their continued growth. The body will then jump up its intake requirement, which will cause the teenager to eat more later on, causing a massive shock to the teenager's system.

This same shock will occur with those who attempt a starvation diet.

Vomiting the recently ingested food is another common method of losing weight. This is a terrible strategy, worse than starvation, simply because of the hydrochloric acid that is released, causing throat and teeth damage.

No worries! There are safe methods to losing your teenage weight. One of the most admirable first steps is to share with friends and family your problem and ask them to assist you.

All of the excellent recommended diet plans are recommended by doctors. There are hundred of them out there, and all tested and proven to work, while focusing on either carbs or proteins, etc.

However, a healthy diet is only healthy if you commit to the right physical activity. With your doctor, work up a great work out plan that will complement your diet.

Dive into playing sports, such as swimming, basketball and football. As a teenager, your body is still designed to withstand rigorous activity.

Despite all the promises made on your local shopping network, there are no fast ways to healthfully lose weight. Commit to a steady diet and physical activity, and if any challenges arise, consult a trained professional.

Fast Weight Loss Diet For Teens

With the current standard of weight loss among our slender Hollywood celebrities, teenagers, being in their influential age, witness this and desire to have the smallest body possible.

Of course, there are thousands of diets that could be rather effective, however you need to make sure you choose a diet that fits your needs, meaning you will remain healthy during and after your diet expires.

Unless you were born into riches and royalty, most diets will thin out more than just your waist. Even though these diets seem practical, the majority will cost more than it took to get you into the shape you are trying to escape from. Since this is the case, perhaps it is time to consider to invent your own diet.

There is no such thing as a diet, only a life style. A life style of a balanced intake and physical activity will give the resources your body needs to live long and healthy. The following are just a few practical tips on how to create your own personal diet, one that is healthy for you.

Meat intake

Meat is a great source of protein, useful in your exercising of muscles; however stir clear of those fatty, red meats. Instead, dive into your white meats, such as chicken or turkey, cutting back on your normal calorie consumption.

A Fruity diet is best

Everything you need can be found in fruits, as they were the original foods of ancient man; all of your needed sources of vitamins and minerals can be found in our everyday fruits. Only certain types of protein are exempt, finding a more excellent source in meats.

Veggies

Fiber, more vitamins and minerals can be found in your greens and yellows. Eating a pure veggie meal once or twice a week might be the ticket to a healthy level of weight loss.

Remember to do some research on to prepare your veggie meal, as some methods of cooking tend to remove the health benefits.

Commitment to Diet and Exercise Routine

Eating well does not secure a victory in weight loss; rather it provides the tools needed in order to achieve victory. You now need to engage in a scheduled time of physical activity. Eating well and a commitment to an exercise routine, without wavering or excuse, is a great way tackle your goal of weight loss.

Healthy Way For Teens To Lose Weight

There is nothing wrong with eating. The problem occurs when the teenager eats too much food that contains fats and sugars which is reason that many become overweight. Studies show that those who are unable to control it want a quick solution. There are quite a few which are not effective and in reality are potentially dangerous.

One example is the vegetarian diet. In essence, there is nothing wrong with however teens who don't know any better have totally removed chicken and meat products from the dish.

Vegetarians believe it or not still need to eat a little meat such as those derived from poultry products and fish. This is because it has the essential nutrients that are needed while a teen is growing up.

Some people tend to forget all that but there is a downside to it. This is because the teenager will have to eat a wide variety of vegetables to compensate for this.

Some teens have tried drinking herbal tea. These products are very similar to laxative pills because the person will frequently be forced to go to the bathroom and get rid of it. Studies have shown that this is unsafe for a teen who will most likely suffer from dehydration or complications in the colon.

Teens are very susceptible to ads seen on television. There are some on the home television shopping network that promise to lose those extra pounds by going on a diet in just two weeks.

These usually focus on a low calorie diet plan. Although there is nothing wrong should this be done for an adult, again, this is harmful for teens. This is because a sudden loss in the calorie intake will prompt the body to take defensive measures and force one to eat a lot later on to compensate of the deficiency.

In fact, the same effects will happen should the teenager even think of going on a starvation diet.

Another unsafe way to lose weight will be vomit out the food that was eaten. This is worse than starving oneself because the body expels hydrochloric acid that burns the throat and the teeth.

So, is there a healthy way for a teen to lose the excess weight? The answer is yes. The first step is admitting to oneself that it has to end and then sharing this problem with members in the family to get the help and support.

Someone may recommend a diet plan that was made by trained professionals and tested by doctors. There are so many to choose from and some focus more on carbs while others put more emphasis on consuming more proteins.

A healthy diet should have a good follow through with the right exercise. There are various workout programs like lifting weights, attending group classes or burning those calories on the treadmill.

There are also other sports such as basketball, football or swimming that the teen can engage especially when the body can still withstand the pressures of rigorous activity.

There is no such a thing as a fast way to lose weight. The only thing that exists is a safe and healthy one that can make this happen. There will be challenges ahead but this can only be achieved with the help of a trained professional.

The Involvement Of Schools In Teen Weight Loss

If you want to help your children lose weight, some changes have to be made. It is becoming more often that we read and hear a lot about the need to lose weight on a daily basis. Now that obesity is being recognized as an increasing problem, losing weight, especially in teens has gained a lot more significance.

Overweight kids have been the product of a "fast food" lifestyle that most families has grown accustomed with. Daily consumption of hamburgers and fries along with other add-on have made it easier for teens to gain more weight and at the same time get less of the essential nutrients that their growing body needs. It is becoming an unhealthy trend that needs to be addressed. It is usually up to the parents to take action.

So what is usually the quick and easy answer to help teenagers as well as adults lose weight? The simple combination of diet and exercise of course. Almost everyone is aware that following a healthy diet and regular exercise are keys to losing and maintaining a healthy weight. No new research is required before you can look into the causes of obesity in teenagers. More than just the fast food, it is also the larger portion sizes, or increasing inactivity that are causing more teens to become overweight.

There is not one single thing that they can easily change and make fewer people overweight. It is usually a combination of diet, exercise and other things that is the successful answer to any weight issues. The big concern is more on how to find the motivation to eat healthier and exercise regularly. This is probably the most difficult part of trying to lose weight. But even if one has the proper motivation to start eating healthier and exercising more often, trying to keep it up becomes an even harder task.

In the case of teenage kids, proper motivation may come from going to school each day. An educational institution that practices and preaches a healthy lifestyle would be more than helpful in keeping the weight of teenage and even younger kids in check. Schools can institute major changes in order to provide kids with healthy meals and regular exercise. Small steps such as banning soda and fruit drinks can help a lot.

There are many ways that a school might help kids in general become healthier. One is by providing real daily physical education requirements that can help make kids more active physically, a break from a sedentary lifestyle that they may be accustomed with at home. A school can also help in an effective weight loss program for kids by offering only healthy foods at school meals. Unhealthy foods or snacks should not be offered as an option for kids who don't want to eat healthy.

Having adequate fitness equipment available to all students can greatly help in motivating kids to become more active. Such equipment should be made available for everyone and not just for those students who are participating in formal sports. Schools can also increase the number of informal sports that kids can play.

This way, kids do not have to be a member of the varsity basketball team in order to enjoy playing basketball at school. Of all of these changes, the program to increase physical education requirements will likely be the most useful in helping kids reach a healthy weight. Such programs can also help them avoid becoming overweight and further help kids build good habits that might stay with them into adulthood.

Supplementing Teen Weight Loss

It is getting easier for teenagers today to put on weight. There are a number of reasons that make this possible. One of them is the popularity of fast food chains as the main source of daily nourishment for most of teenagers.

To say the least, the kind of food that such establishments provide can really be fattening. And they can not provide the kind of balanced nourishment required by growing teens. But sad to say, in this generation of convenience and busier lifestyle, fast food chains have become an ideal choice especially for the parents who might not find the time to prepare meals for their children.

When you realize that your teen is getting fatter and putting up more and more weight, you have to act early in order to prevent it from getting worse. An overweight teen can easily acquire a number of life threatening conditions such as high blood pressure, diabetes and increased risk of strokes. Early action would usually help in preventing such conditions from developing in your child as he or she grows. There are a numbor of solutions available to help your lose that excess weight.

You can put your overweight teen on a diet to help him or her get rid of that excess weight. A healthy diet combined with regular exercise is essential to a healthy way of losing weight. You can also give him or her weight loss supplements that will further help in maintaining a healthy means of getting rid of that excess weight. One of the supplements that your teen can possibly take is calcium.

Most people are not aware that weight loss diets may sometimes affect the amount of nutrients that the body gets. Some diets may promise quick weight loss but may not be giving the body with the essential nutrients that it needs, especially the bones. Calcium and other nutrients are sometimes in low supply during periods of dieting which may lead to increased chances of developing conditions such as osteoporosis.

Parents should be aware that dieting may lead to a low supply in calcium in their teens. They should be able to provide their children with a variety of calcium and other supplements so that the dieting teens would still be getting all the essential nutrients they need to grow and develop.

And not only that, essential nutrients such as calcium may even aid your teenager in losing excess weight. There have been numerous studies that show that calcium may help in reducing body fat.

The reason for this is because calcium is a known fat burner. Diets with a healthy amount of calcium seem to favor burning rather than storing fat in the body. Calcium in the body is stored in fat cells and this plays an important role in fat storage and breakdown. Calcium may be able to change the efficiency of losing weight. Further studies have shown that dieters with the highest overall calcium intake experience losing more weight, and the people with the lowest calcium intake had the highest percentage of body fat.

When overall calorie consumption is taken into consideration, it not only helps keep a person's weight in check, but it can also be associated specifically with substantial decreases in body fat. A low daily calcium intake is associated with greater tendency to gain weight, particularly in adolescent girls and adult women.

What You Need To Know About Teen Weight Loss

In world where physical comeliness matters, more and more people are giving too much emphasis on physical appearance. They are becoming interested—even obsessed—in using so many products and services that can help them improve their physical appearance.

Today, one of the biggest problems of people—especially by teenagers all over the world—is being overweight or obesity. Too much weight—caused by overeating and lack of exercise—is becoming one of the problems especially of teenagers that cause them to lose confidence.

If you are a parent who has an obese or overweight child and you would want to help him or her to lose weight safe and effectively, here are some steps that you can do:

1. Help your child to come up with a great decision. Losing weight is a decision you must help your child with. The first thing that you can do is to talk to your child. Ask him or her what he or she thinks about herself. If he or she confesses that he/she doesn't feel good about his or her physical appearance, then its now time to ask your child what he/she wants to do.

Give your child suggestions on how he/she improve herself. Ask him or her if he or she is willing to lose weight and help your child all the way. Once you and your child have made a decision, start plotting your plan on how to lose weight effectively, safely, and the healthy way. Aside from making the major decision whether to lose or nor to lose weight, the decision must also include the full participation of both parties in the agenda.

Aside from assuring your child that that he or she has your full support, it would also be a wise decision if you both formulate a specific plan how you are going to approach this endeavor. The decision will also include the possible resources and strategies you can use.

2. If possible, try to change your eating and exercising patterns together. If you really want to help your child lose weight, you should try formulating an eating and exercise plan that can help him or her lose weight effectively. An effective plan may include eating foods low in fat and low in sugar along with a great deal of regular exercise.

3. Look for nonprofessional support weight loss programs and use them if you can.
Today, there are two weight loss programs that most experts recommend: the TOPS or Take
Off Pounds Sensibly which is a self-help club encourages parent-child participation and the
Weight Watchers. Statistics say that most people who enroll in these programs drop out even
before the program ends, so it is very important for parents to guide their children so they won't
give up easily.

***4. Ask help from professionals and experts that have expertise in cognitive-behavior
therapy and weight.*** Since obesity is one of the major problems of teenagers, more and more
psychologists offer their services to help people who are overweight to lose weight.

***5. Send your child to high-quality weight loss camps or to residential weight loss
programs.*** Losing weight can be traumatic experience for your child. Giving him or her a fresh
new environment to start with can help him or her a lot to pursue the weigh loss endeavor.

Today, there are so many weight loss camps created specifically for those children who would
want to lose weight away from the eyes of people who are eagerly and intently watching him or
her. In the first few weeks of your child in this new task, he or she may find it hard to
concentrate because of the pressure given by the people and the environment. You can help
him or her if you look for a safe and clinically appropriate environment that can help her or him
focus on losing weight.

Weight Loss Plan For Teens

Studies have shown that there are a lot of people who are either obese or overweight. People can blame it on the food being served in the cafeteria or the type of meals being served in the fast food joint but in the end, the only one to blame is the person.

This is because everyone has a choice whether to live with a good diet plan or not and those who are too heavy just decided to eat more than what is allowable.

Luckily, there is a way to stop this from getting any worse. There are doctors and dietitians that the teen can go up to help create a weight loss plan.

Is there one plan out there suitable for every teen? The answer is no. This will depend on the physical condition of the patient after an examination has been conducted.

One of the advantages of losing weight while the person is still young is that there are not that limitations compared to an adult. This allows the body to burn calories much faster when engaging in a workout or playing a certain sport.

Since physical education class is not enough to get those calories, the doctor can recommend that the patient work out in the gym or in the youth center. These places have the equipment such as treadmills, weights and other sports facilities that can cater to the weight loss plan.

Most people are advised to engage in a physical activity for 20 minutes three times a week. Teens have a lot of energy and it wouldn't hurt to do this everyday. Since the body may adapt to the changes, the doctor may recommend some variations to help those extra pounds weekly.

The chances of getting the desired weight will not happen if the food being consumed is not being monitored. The dietitian must also come up with a program in order for this work.

The basic dietary plan is called the no nonsense balanced diet. This means simply getting enough carbohydrates, proteins and fats in each meal because there are many who put more emphasis on one or the other.

Having too much carbohydrates could be the cause for someone being overweight. This can be stopped by following a low carb diet plan where the patient will have to cut down on carbohydrates and replace this with food that is rich in proteins and fats. People will see results in less than a month and just have to continue to maintain the ideal weight.

Another option is the low calorie diet in which the teen will eat six small meals a day instead of the three that people normally practice. This is distributed during different hours of the day and is proven to works in just 14 days.

Aside from exercising and dieting, the weight loss plan involves getting enough rest. This will allow the body to recharge from the activities of the day to be prepared for the challenges tomorrow.

Overweight teens will not lose the excess pounds overnight. The teen can only make this happen by following the doctor's advice with regards to the food being consumed and with proper exercise.

One way to check on the effectiveness of the plan will be to go up the weighing scale. If it is not working as projected, perhaps the teen can ask for another weight loss plan given there are different ways that can make this happen.

Dieting with a Busy Schedule

While adopting a dieting routine, the most commonly quoted problem is lack of sufficient time to prepare the correct meals for our dietary requirements. It is obviously easier to throw something into the pot or hit a fast food stand rather than cook a healthy, nutritious and balanced meal that we ought to be consuming.

There are certain tips that one can follow to control the urge to go off track, and make sure you are always strictly following your diet plans. The first one is by cooking once a week. Using this method, you prepare enough food to last you for an entire week, on a specific day. So, you have a meal that is diet friendly for every night in that week. If the rest of your family is also incorporating your dieting plans, this method can be applied in such cases too. Adopting healthy eating habits and planning a balanced diet routine for your entire family is an excellent way to teach your children, and at the same time, it keeps you motivated and helps you fight temptation.

By adopting the once a week cooking method, you have to freeze food that will not be consumed immediately and thaw it when you decide to cook the evening meal after you return from work. This process works perfectly irrespective of how many dance practices, band recitals and soccer games that you have on that week's schedule. Thus, you can follow your diet program and also provide a great and healthy supper for your family, every single night of the week.

Always make sure that you have sufficient quantity of clean and fresh fruits, vegetables and suitable salad ingredients, so that these dishes are easily accessible for quick lunches. If these dishes are easily available, it will help you in fighting the temptation to have a high calorie meal. It will also ensure that you have your daily serving of fresh, nutritious fruits and vegetables.

You can also keep some packaged yoghurt or low calorie pudding cups as a quick and ready to eat dairy product. Efficient planning and preparation is essential if you want to achieve your weight reduction goals. By making the food much ahead of the stipulated time, you will not miss out on the convenience of high calorie, packaged foods that many of us thrive on when we are not dieting.

Another useful way to save time is to use opportunities and apply your fitness plans during the course of the day. Instead of performing a lengthy exercise every day, try and bring a few fitness activities into your day. (Climb stairs during lunch hour, park you car at the top level so that you will have to take the stairs), park far away from the mall entrance and check if there is a clear walking path! You will be fascinated by the amount of hidden opportunities that are available to bring your fitness program into a normally busy day. The challenge lies, not in finding time, but in finding the hidden activities. Dieting does not have to be as tedious and time consuming as it appears to be. There are plenty of pre packaged diet plans for people who wish to adopt a diet plan, if you feel that it may be the best option for you. Whether you are planning to take up Weight Watchers frozen foods, or Lean Cuisine meals, Jenny Craig, or Slim Fast program, enumerable opportunities are available to combine dieting and fitness even into an extremely busy schedule. Remember to keep these tips in mind while planning your diet routine.

Dieting And Fitness

If one wants to live a long, healthy lifestyle, there are two essential ingredients, namely, diet and fitness. Some believe that these two factors mean one and the same, but the truth is they are a lot different. It is possible however to have an extremely healthy diet with bad fitness levels. Similarly, one may be physically fit but may follow an unbalanced dieting program.

There is a clever line in the song "Fruitcakes" by Jimmy Buffet, when his 'lady' grieves
"I treat my body like a temple
You treat yours like a tent"

I just can't avoid thinking about this line when I observe people around the globe, who keep adopting crazy diet plans with the hope of achieving weight loss like those who market the product.

Truthfully speaking, one can lose weight through effective diet plans alone, but it is a difficult process. One can be maintain physical fitness and still be a little on the heavier side. Our lifestyle is largely dependent on the kind of food we consume. If our diet plan has high fat and low substance products, our bodies will lack the necessary fuel to burn excess fat. Similarly, if we don't give our bodies the tools required to build muscles, the number of weights we lift is of no significance.

In order to produce best results related to a healthy lifestyle, diet and fitness must work hand in hand. Your fitness regime must burn the excess fat and calories while a healthy diet must supply the fuel and nutrients necessary to build muscle. I have often heard that a pound of fat weighs more than the same amount of muscle. Though this is not completely true, we know that a pound of muscle will occupy less area in the body when compared to a pound of fat. Talking in terms of pounds, I would prefer mine to be made of muscle rather than fat. Throughout your efforts, you must keep in mind that dieting alone will not build muscle.

You must realize that, in the process of adding muscles, you may be losing weight without showing significant progress on the weighing scale. It is essential that you remember this throughout the weight reduction program. If you measure progress by relying on the scales, you will be misled to a large extent. Many people do not realize this, and tend to give up due to frustration, while they are actually beginning to make progress. Do not let yourself be misled by the weighing scale. Look in to the mirror, wear a pair of tight pants, and then measure your waist. Don't measure your weight loss success by checking how many pounds you lost this week, instead, see how it feels after climbing a few floors.

By merging your diet routine with your fitness regime, you help the body to lose any extra fat that may have been consumed. You can use this trick to make up for your tiny urges. All you have to do is burn off the extra calories by working out a little more than the usual. It is better to avoid doing this frequently, but occasionally using this "cheat" is fairly acceptable as it will not produce any mammoth effect on your diet plan.

One must look at diet plans and fitness programs as a simple ball and glove relationship. Though it is possible to play ball without using the glove, it works better when you use both. When diet and fitness are combined effectively, it will produce excellent weight loss results to people who take both seriously. The important thing to be remembered here is that neither will work well alone, and they will not work at all unless you are serious, focused and willing to put in every ounce of effort. You must give it a high priority in your daily lifestyle, so that you can achieve fantastic results.

Eating Healthy On Vacation

You may find it difficult to resist the urge to abandon your healthy eating habits when you are on vacation. Though you may be determined to stick to your dieting principles, it is highly possible that you may get carried away and tends to buy an ice cream now and then. There are certain ways to keep a watch over what you eat on vacation.

Nowadays, it is so very easy to ask for a vegetarian or a low calorie meal on airplanes. But if you decide to drive to your holiday spot, finding healthy eating options may turn out to be a bit difficult.

Instead of depending on greasy meals for your daily nutrition, just pack some healthy alternatives in a cooler with ice packs. Sandwiches, fruits, vegetables, crackers and yoghurt are great options to carry with you on your road trip.

When you arrive at the hotel, you could do yourself good by turning down the mini bar key - it helps fight temptation. If the hotel offers you a continental breakfast option, choose cereals, fruits and protein. If the hotel provides a stove, you could consider carrying your own nutritious meal with you.

But if you have no option but to eat outside, make sure you do so only at times when you are really hungry. Some restaurants tend to serve large quantities, so watch out and remember to cut down on your next meal if you over do it.

If you are unable to eat three square meals, try to divide it into six smaller meals, because your body requires fuel almost once every four hours. While eating out, try to avoid appetizers. But always make sure never to skip a meal.

Whenever possible, avoid eating large portions of food at night. When your body slows down and prepares for sleep, the calorie burning process takes place at a slower rate. Never consume bread before going to bed, and ensure that you avoid the butter. Instead, choose poultry or fish as your meal, with a vegetable side dish.

Though its may sound difficult, sticking to your healthy eating habits on vacation is not as tough as it sounds. All you need is a little will power to fight the urge to go for foods that aren't good for you. Therefore, you will enjoy a healthy lifestyle through healthy eating.

Always keep in mind that healthy eating is important. Though you may give in to cravings at times, do not make it a habit. A single pizza or an ice cream cone is acceptable provided you know your limit.

Weight Loss Surgery

All who are looked at to be very obese have only a few options to lose weight when time period is very critical. Most have shifted from one kind of diet to another for a major part of their lives but only to realize failure and also develop a sense of helplessness and hopelessness which in turn leads to a very pessimistic approach in life.

The general misconception about the over obese people is that they were solely responsible and if they chose otherwise they wouldn't be this fat. This is only a nice in theory but not true in practice generally. There are some medical conditions that cause certain bodily dysfunctions and hence these people can't control weight they put on. There are environmental issues as well which can influence the weight as well. But it's ironic that many cases who are drug addicts and alcoholics are cared for and seen with better compassion than a person who is obese.

Surgery itself is big surgery and isn't an option that can be taken carelessly without thought. Many people realize that surgery involves a big change in their lifestyle also a new method of eating which is a lifetime commitment. Due to these facts it's suggested that all those getting the surgery must have a BMI greater than at least 40. This in turn means that it's advised for guys who are more than a hundred pound extra and women who have extra bulk of eighty pounds or so.

One should carefully consider benefits and risks of such a surgery prior to deciding that surgery is the plan of action you are taking. Risks involved are great and must not be overlooked by desperation to reduce weight .Nutrition based deficiencies result in 20% of people who have opted for this surgery as the end result in insufficiency of nutrients. This may cause osteoporosis and worse conditions as you grow old. Some complications result from surgery by itself. You will have lifetime issues when eating a lot or the incorrect kinds of food, and some who reach the goals find out that weight can come back at times. Like life itself, there is no assurance about weight loss surgeries.

To decide whether or not you need this surgery , you should ask yourself some of the following queries which may help make up your mind in either way.

Is my extra bulk hampering significant daily activities?

Is my extra bulk causing any other condition which may harm my well being?
Is my extra bulk something I feel I should control by myself?
Will I be able to handle consequences and all the follow ups that are required?

The main problem with many people who need to resort to surgery is the fact that they can't take control of the body again. The chances of a candidate for surgery getting rid of the fat by his own methods are very less as he is most likely to have tried and also failed every other diet given in any book.

You can only decide if or not surgery is a good option for your needs. But if you finally decide that's what you want to do, then discuss all possible consequences clearly with your doctor in order to avoid the possibility of any serious damage later on during your older years.

The Dark Side Of Fad Diets

Many people are surprised that fad diets aren't recommended when they appear to produce good results. There are many websites on the internet which claim to provide effective weight reduction in very few days. This kind of weight reduction is temporary. It is almost 90% water which returns to your body when it gets hydrated again, which happen otherwise cause severe health complications.

Some other fad diets which are less prominent crash diets, have outrageous claims and are just over hyped. They tend to be effective for some time, and is usually huge money making venture for its inventor in product sales. In some best cases, there are good diet programs which will help you achieve your weight loss goals, but you may have been able to get that from your doctor, for free. In worst cases, these fad diets will prove to be too difficult to follow and you will abandon them after a week.

Disadvantages of Fad Diets

1. Fad Diets, which promise fast and easy weight reduction, are normally based on consuming more of a certain food type and none of others. In this way, you will not obtain the benefits of a balanced diet. You are sometimes recommended to take supplements, but some of these supplements are not taken by the body, unless they are consumed along with food that your diet has removed. After a couple of weeks, you will start developing deficiency due to malnutrition.

2. Often, Fad diets are boring and involve many restrictions. The enthusiasm of the idea will vanish after a day or two, following which your cravings will increase and make you break the diet. Finally, it may make you feel guilty that you were not strictly following the diet.

3. Most of these fad diets don't follow the instructions given by the American Heart Association and other such bodies for nutrition levels in food. These diets may suggest high fat and low carbohydrate foods which will ultimately result in heart problems. They may say that the diet should be followed only on a short term basis. But if you don't achieve your goal plan by then, you will either tend to continue with an unhealthy plan, or stop and regain the weight you lost.

4. Most fad diets don't supply your body with the necessary amount of fresh fruits and vegetables and your diet program does not give you the diverse food supplements that you require.

5. Weight loss programs that are quick are only temporary, short lived solutions and will not have any permanent effect on your eating habits. Producing permanent change is the only solution to remain at the targeted weight once you have reached it. Fad diets are yo-yo cycles of quick weight reduction and equally rapid weight gain. Such an effect is bad for your health as well as your self esteem and you would have been better off staying overweight.

No matter what the publicity materials say, fad diets will not assist you on a long term basis. The ideal way to produce sustained weight loss is by eating a varied and properly balanced diet, avoiding high calorie foods, exercising regularly and most importantly, by avoiding fad diets.

Free Weight Loss Programs

More and more people are adapting their lifestyles to strict fitness regimes. While some do it to acquire a sexy new body, some do it as they are embarrassed with their present self, and some others do it just to remain healthy and fit. There are plenty of fitness routines available on the internet, in spas and gyms. Some of these programs are very expensive and heavy on the pocket. One may lose weight by simply trying to manipulate the necessary finance to adopt these fitness routines.

One need not visit the gym and the spa and spend hours working out and performing strenuous exercises in order to obtain that beautiful, sexy body. Several books available at bookstores offer effective and convenient weight reduction programs for free, although the books don't come for free. These programs are gaining a lot of popularity through much hype, publicity and reviews which often confuse the person as to which one he must follow. Before you choose a weight loss program, go through these summaries about popular diet programs.

The first book is Dr. Atkins' New Diet Revolution. This program endorses high protein and low carbohydrate foods. One may thrive on meat and vegetables but must completely avoid pasta and bread. There are no restrictions on fat, so you can indulge on the salad dressing, while spreading the butter freely. However, this diet lacks fiber and calcium content and limited composition of grain and fruits, while it is high in fat.

The next review is Dr. Heller's Carbohydrate Addict's Diet. This diet program incorporates low carbohydrate foods in the diet. It allows consumption of vegetables, fruits, meat, grains and dairy products. It advocates consumption of fewer carbohydrates. The "Reward" meal is very high in fats.

Dr. Goor's Choose to Lose imposes restriction on consuming fatty foods. The person is provided with a "fat" budget and is allowed to spend it. There is no pressure on carbohydrate intake. It allows consumption of meat, poultry and low-fat dairy products. It advocates intake of fruits, vegetables, bread, pasta and grains. This program is reasonably healthy as it supplies sufficient amount of fruits, veggies and saturated fat. However, one must monitor triglyceride levels. If it is high, cut down on carbohydrate and indulge on unsaturated fats.

The next summary is the DASH Diet. It encourages intake of moderate quantities of unsaturated fat and protein and high carbohydrate foods. It is basically aimed at lowering blood pressure, and it follows the pyramid guide. Hence, it advocates high intake of grains, fruits, vegetables and low-fat foods. However, some people feel that it involves excessive eating to produce a significant loss in weight.

The following summary is about Dr. Ornish's Eat More, Weigh Less. It advocates vegetarian and low-fat foods. It restricts "glow" foods and recommends a watch over egg whites and non-fat dairy. But this diet is deficient in calcium and restrains intake of poultry and seafood.

Eat Right for your Type. This is interesting because it recommends the diet based on the dieter's blood group. It encourages plenty of meat intakes for people with O type blood. But the diet plans for certain other blood types are not balanced and are very low in calories. Besides, there is no recorded proof that blood group varies the dietary requirements.

The Pritkin Principle

It focuses on cutting down the calories by eating watery foods that tend to satisfy hunger. Intake of fruits, vegetables, pasta, oatmeal, salads, low-fat dairy and soups are allowed. It limits protein rich foods to seafood and poultry. Though it is healthy as it provides less saturated fat, it is low in calcium and lean protein content.

Volumetrics

Advises low calorie food intake. Its recommendations are similar to Pitkin but it asks the dieter to refrain from eating dry foods like crackers, pretzels and popcorn. It is reasonably healthy as it has high supplies in fruits, vegetables and also in low calorie, unsaturated fats.

The Zone

It has moderately low carbohydrate content and high protein content. This advocates low-fat and protein rich foods like fish, chicken, veggies, grains and fruits. Though it is healthy, it lacks in calcium.

Weight Watchers

It is high in carbohydrate content, and moderate on proteins and fats. It is a very healthy plan and is extremely flexible. It gives the dieter the liberty to follow his own diet plan than restrict him to a pre-packaged routine.

Atkins Diet Basics

The Atkins diet has become quite an old trend now though it has become a recognized fact among the health conscious as well as the dieters. Dr. Atkins's New Diet Revolution book discovered a whole new bunch of audience who had problems with low-fat diet plans. However, we cannot say that everyone surrounded by this hype is familiar with the fundamental principles of this diet plan.

Here are the important principles based on which the Atkins diet has been designed for giving best results. The theory of the diet deals with why fats get accumulated in our body. As per the study conducted by Dr. Atkins, too much consumption of simple sugars and carbohydrates would lead to weight gain. In this regard, your waistline plays a vital role in the sense that more than the calories and the quantity of fat we consume; it is the manner in which the carbohydrates are processed, which matters. A phenomenon termed "insulin resistance" has been explained by D. Atkins in this regard. He says that the main reason for many people being overweight is because of improper working of the cells in their bodies.

Sugar levels tend to get elevated when too much of carbohydrates and sugar is consumed in turn resulting in insulin being released from the pancreas. This happens because it is necessary for storing sugar in the form of glycogen in the muscle cells and liver which is used later on when extra energy is needed. But, glycogen can be stored only to a certain extent after which it is converted into fat. Anyone who consumes too much of carbohydrates tend to face such a situation.

On the other hand, individuals who are insulin resistant face tougher problems in storing and using the excess carbohydrates consumed by them. Higher the level of insulin, higher is the resistance. When the cells try to fight against the increasing level of insulin, they end up producing more of fat and lesser amount of glycogen. The result of this is extra weight gain in insulin resistant individuals.

Insulin resistant people have many more problems to face which includes fatigue, low blood sugar (resulting in hypoglycaemia), brain fogging (loss of creativity, poor memory and inability to focus), depression, high blood sugar and sleepiness.

A diet constrained in carbohydrates is the only solution for individuals who are insulin resistant. The bottom line followed by the Atkins diet is restriction of intake of carbohydrates in all forms. Sodas, sweets and cookies which come under simple sugars, complex carbohydrates like grains, rice and bread are restricted under the Atkins diet. Wholesome carbohydrates like brown rice, whole wheat bread and oatmeal are also restricted under the diet plan.

The diet restricts the intake of carbohydrate to an amount below 40 grams per day which would in turn bring the body to a state of ketosis resulting in fats being burnt as fuel to provide energy. This would put off more insulin production in the body and the already stored fat would be burnt to provide energy, the end result being weight loss.

An added advantage of this diet plan is that, it will put an end to the carbohydrate cravings. A high carbohydrate diet is never fulfilling to a person as we can never get enough of it. On the other hand, with a constraint on the amount of carbohydrate to be consumed, we come over the craving for gradually with the passage of time.

The Atkins program, though strict in the earlier stages, in the longer run enriches us in properly balancing our diet. The diet can be used slowly according to the individual necessity and a perfect balance between carbohydrate use and health can be achieved y reintroducing little amounts of carbohydrates.

The primary principle of this diet program has helped in formulating several other low-carbohydrate diet plans. However, for the insulin resistant people, the most satisfying diet plan is the renowned Atkins diet plan!

Getting More Alkaline Into Your Diet

The PH miracle diet has revolutionized the perspective on eating. The diet aspires to achieve ph levels of 20% acid and 80% alkaline in food intake. This aims at equaling the ph levels of the bloodstream, which bends towards the alkaline. This can be challenging for quite a few people, as the food they usually tend to indulge in is considered mostly acidic. It thus becomes important to recognize sources of alkaline content, construct a list of such foods and add them to your PH miracle diet.

Alkalizing foods neutralize the acidity present in the bloodstream, thereby giving the body a sensation of rejuvenation. They regenerate and restore cells in the system and refresh the body, thus acting as a "breath of fresh air". Repeated intake of food high in acid content causes premature break down of the body. These "acid bombs" are carried throughout the system by the bloodstream, causing harm and posing a threat and danger to the body. We can optimize the PH level in our blood by identifying what foods have an alkalizing property, and integrating it in our diet in higher amounts. Levels 7 and greater are considered alkaline, the levels of human blood being between 7.35-7.45.

The simplest way to get alkaline into the system is by eating fruits and vegetables. Some alkalizing vegetables are: barley grass, alfalfa, beet greens, beets, carrots, cabbage, broccoli, chard greens, cauliflower, celery, collard greens, dandelions, cucumber, green beans, garlic, egg plant, green peas, kohlrabi, kale, lettuce, mustard greens, onions, nightshade veggies, peppers, peas, parsnip, radishes, pumpkin, rutabaga, spinach, sea veggies, sweet potato, sprouts, watercress, tomato, wild greens and what grass.

Some alkalizing fruits are: avocados, apricots, apples, berries, bananas, blackberries, cherries, cantaloupe, coconut, cherries, currants, figs, dates, grapes, honeydew, grapefruit, limes, lemons, muskmelons, oranges, nectarines, peaches, pineapple, pears, raspberries, raisins, strawberries, rhubarb, tangerines, strawberries, tropical fruits, tomatoes and watermelon.

In the process of addition of more alkaline in ones diet, protein can pose a problem. All animal derived protein is acidic. But there are proteins that are alkalizing. Some are almonds, millet, chestnuts, tofu, whey protein powder and tempeh.

What is food without those herbs, spices and sweeteners, which add greatly to its character? These alkalizing embellishments can be added to your culinary endeavors to balance out the PH levels. Condiments which have an alkalizing effect are: curry, cinnamon, ginger, chili pepper, mustard, sea salt, miso, stevia, tamari and all herbs.

Minerals are also essential for health. Proper blood PH balance can be maintained by identifying which minerals are alkalizing. Some are: potassium, cesium, sodium, magnesium and calcium.

In addition to these, there are some ingredients that make the addition of alkaline to the diet even easier. These may be listed as: vinegar, apple cider, alkaline antioxidant water, lecithin granules, bee pollen, probiotic cultures, molasses, green juices, soured dairy products, fresh fruit juices, veggie juices, and mineral water.

Knowledge of which foods and which supplements add alkaline to the PH levels is just the first step. Implementation, which takes commitment and planning is the next. The best way to test the body's PH level, once these foods have been added to the diet, is the saliva strip test. These tests are available in most of the health food stores. A PH between 7 and 8 boasts of good health.

One should not forget that the aim of the PH miracle diet is to ensure that acidic intake is less than the alkaline intake. This does not necessarily mean that one cannot consume foods that are more acidic. The balance of ones diet should merely be geared towards alkaline foods. Maintaining an appropriate PH balance, one can ensure that the body performs at an optimum level.

Shopping Tips For The Ph Miracle Diet

There are a few guidelines to be followed if you are all set to experiment with the astounding pH diet plan. The first thing to be taken care of is to clean up all the food stuff with high acidic content out of the refrigerator and the pantry. However, this would become difficult if you stay with other people in the house. In such a state, you need to take care that you clear out food stuff which tempts you the most.

Natural food stores and health stores are great options to get the food stuff you will be consuming during the diet period though grocery stores would also be suitable to get the needful things. In case you are in an area without such kind of specialty stores, the local grocery is the best solution.

Certain points which need to be kept in mind while shopping as per your diet requirements are discussed here. Make a list of the items that you need to purchase. It is no use walking around the store trying to recollect everything that you need. You can also plan the week's menu which you would be following and shop according to it. This would help you in buying only the stuff that you need and would therefore save time, money and wastage of items. You will have to buy a lot of alkaline stuff which would mainly be from a variety of vegetables.

The next thing to be taken care of is that you need to be on a complete alkaline diet when you initially start off with the pH diet. Every kind of the pH diet, whether strict or lenient aims at a perfect balance between alkaline and acids. Hence, this should be kept in mind while preparing grocery lists and menus. Food stuff with lower levels of acids consists of whole grain pasta, bananas, eggs, dried beans, wheat bread, nuts and milk. A proportion of 70 percent alkaline to 30 percent acids is considered ideal.

While at a grocery store, you will notice that you would be more on the outside sections of the store as that is the area which generally comprises of fresh food items which may match your needs during the diet period. The outer rim invariably consists of farm fresh products, meat and/or deli products and the dairy products.

Vegetables are the most prominent components of the pH diet and hence more focus would be on them while shopping. Frozen and conventional produce contribute nothing to the diet plan and hence it is an absolute waste using them. Instead, opt for farm fresh produce if you can afford to get it.

Another thing to be avoided is canned vegetables and fruits. They are absolutely unhealthy as they have a negative effect on the alkalinity of the fruits and vegetables and they also contain a great deal of sodium in them. If fresh produce cannot be purchased, it is better to go with frozen ones.

The best way to shop is by purchasing equal or balanced amounts of acidic and alkaline food stuff so that you can get used to the new way of eating as well as living. Just being extremely strict about the diet you consume will not produce the desired results. Rather, start gradually and balance food items in such a way that you get rid of all the acidic food in your diet with the passage of the period of diet plan.

The "Quick Weight Loss Diet" Trend Disadvantage

There is nothing unusual in getting frustrated or feeling guilty or feeling worse about not fitting into a smaller size dress even after a month of hard work through a rapid weight loss program. This is because; sometimes things which we think would motivate would actually backfire.

It is therefore advisable to set more easily achievable targets for oneself. Hence, in case you are going to apply the new-clothes technique, decrease the size gradually and do not burn a hole in your pocket by buying expensive clothes with a hope of losing weight in a very short span of time. One more thing to be kept in mind is that if you continuously repent not losing weight quickly, you tend to end up slipping in rapid weight loss plans and fad diets.

One bitter but true fact is that there is no single diet plan which has been proved to aid in rapid loss of weight and there are no swift ways for people to lose weight more than what their body can actually provide for. Such diets can never be effective in the longer run.

What Works Best

Since the apt attitude and the correct principle are not applied, all these fad diets and swift weight loss programs do not prove efficient and effective. This ends up in weight gain after a certain period of time which would make the person feel even worse.

Such quick fixes for losing weight are termed fad diets as they are nothing more than a trend, a fad. People would realize this only when they see that the diet has not helped them in any way.

The points discussed below are the things to be considered before blindly trusting the so called effective weight losing programs that are being promoted in the markets after spending so many bucks. They are just namesake stories to make people prefer their diet programs. So, here they go:-

1. Missing out on meals

A diet program can be definitely termed fad diet if it calls for the individual to skip meals at any time of the day. Not eating food at proper time may lead to serious hitches especially if the person is diabetic.

Skipping meals is completely unhealthy as it would only result in low blood sugar, otherwise known as hypoglycaemia which would result in more consumption of food in the upcoming meals.

2. Dieting Devoid Of Exercise Or The Vice-Versa

Exercises are very important for maintaining a healthy and fit body. It helps in maintaining proper circulation of blood in the body as well as in carrying out other processes.
Thus, diet plans which are void of exercises are basically pointless and useless. For proper maintenance of the body, diet and exercise must be combined together in the right proportion.

3. Dawdling Continuously

Postponing diet plans is not the best thing to be done. This is because postponement would lead to lethargy. If the diet plan calls for you to lose weight within a stipulated time, it clearly implies that it is nothing but a wannabe trend setting fad diet which is absolutely unhealthy.

Precisely, we can say that slowly losing the excess weight by proper diet and exercise is a better way to lose weight than just blindly following a so called rapid fad diet which might result in more complications and side-effects. It is said so because a fad diet may not make the individual feel good about the whole process while the process of planned and healthy weight loss may make him feel great as well as leave behind a positive enthusiasm.

Lose Weight The Herbal Way

Nowadays, several obese Americans have the need to shed those extra pounds. Staying fit would help them lead a healthy lifestyle and also remove the load off their body, improving their all round well being.

There are several dieting options which one can adopt. Some are fitness equipment, exercise programs, dietary supplements, dietary foods, drinks and soaps which apparently help you reduce weight as you bathe.

Another option that remains open to shed those extra pounds is to adopt herbal methods.

For people who wish to lose weight naturally, herbal weight reduction products are their best bet. But when one takes herbal supplements to procure weight loss, the waiting period is longer due to the mild effect of pills which come from natural herbs and plant life.

Below are a few herbal weight reduction options that you can take a look at:

1. Herbal Weight Loss Product

There are plenty of products in the market, which help you to lose weight herbally. Even on the internet you will find many such herbal weight reduction medicines.

But you must be careful about the products you choose because though some claim to be natural and safe; they cause side effects on the long run because of insufficient research on the long term effects of these herbal products.

Listed below are some chemical ingredients that are used in herbal products which you must carefully avoid as they may produce a harmful effect to your body's health.

> Senna. It is herbal laxative, and is the prime ingredient used in weight reduction teas. It is stimulated in the colon. The major drawback of Senna is dehydration, colon disorder and even addiction. When addiction occurs, some people find it difficult to perform bowel movements in the absence of this herb.

> ***Chromium picolinate.*** It is a synthetic ingredient used in herbal products. Chromium helps in regulation of the level of blood sugar. However, excessive consumption may damage the chromosomes, and in some cases, leads to dehydration of the body.

> ***St. John's wort.*** It increases chemical production in the brain. But if it is used incorrectly, it causes sensitivity in the skin and eye region, fatigue, gastrointestinal disorder and itching.

Though most herbal products say that they are 100% natural and safe, one must carefully study the ingredients and effects of the products before taking up these dietary capsules.

2. Organic Food

Organic food has worked its way into hotels and houses in Wichita, Kansas. People who consume organic food strongly believe that eating organic food helps their body and the environment simultaneously.

People who eat organically produced eggs and vegetables say that they are way healthier and save a lot of money that is usually spent on doctors and medicines. This is an extremely good option for weight watchers too as they don't add much weight to your body when compared to food products that are processed chemically.

3. Green Tea

Recent research reveals that drinking green tea or extracts of green tea helps in burning excess calories. Green tea with caffeine is found to increase fat loss by about 40%, thereby reducing the fat content rapidly.

This is a very good option for people who wish to reduce weight. On conducting experiments, it has been discovered that people who consumed green tea had lost 2 to 3 times more weight compared to those who did not.

Thus, green tea is an obvious, natural option for people who wish to treat obesity. It also serves as a healthy dietary option and has extremely good effects on the body when compared to caffeine foods. A cup of green tea provides an immediate surge of energy without carrying the side effects produced by caffeine products.

3. Caffeine

Drinking coffee gives the body a much needed energy boost and also helps to increase the fat burning. It increases the energy in the body, consequently increasing the rate at which fat is burnt.

4. Immortality Herb

Its biological name is Gymnostemna Pentaphyllum and it has the following advantages:

> Increased Fat burning rate
> Increases blood flow
> Maintains healthy blood pressure
> Reduces artery blocks

5. Cider Vinegar

There are many pills and supplements which contain apple cider vinegar as its primary ingredient. Its benefits include:

> Controls blood pressure
> Improves cholesterol level
> Aids weight loss
> Helps in prevention of rheumatoid arthritis

Low Carbohydrate Diet

With the publicity of Atkins' diet, low carbohydrate diets have become the latest trend in recent years. Weight reduction has become everyone's aim and they are looking for quick and simple options to lose weight. In some cases, people who not need to lose weight get overly stressed when they gain a few pounds. In certain other cases, people may have to shed pounds to solve medical complications and may possess more than a hundred pounds that they need to get rid of.

There are several different diet plans available, including low carbohydrate diets and truthfully speaking, all of them will prove successful in weight loss provided they are followed strictly. This does not necessarily imply that one must follow the diet requirements each and every second of the day. The essential point is to stir clear of occasions where you feast and indulge on foods that are banned in your diet plan. If you are able to pull this off and stick to the diet plan without much difficulty, you will emerge successful. Almost everyone has one of these days - the challenge lies in letting them go and taking them as another successful step on the path to permanent weight reduction.

It is important to adopt a diet plan that is easy for you to follow. Low carbohydrate diet is the most popular dieting option as its rules are fairly simple. As the title suggests, it involves limited intake of carbohydrate rich foods. This includes pasta, bread, grains, rice and potatoes. Sugar intake also accounts for carbohydrate consumption. It is easy to avoid these carbohydrate rich foods once their composition is understood.

The main point of criticism when it comes to low carbohydrate dieting is that dieters get most of their calories from dairy, meat and other fat rich substances. This may lead to rise in cholesterol levels and other problems which arise due to high consumption of saturated fat. It is recommended that you take medical advice before adopting such a diet plan. In some cases, weight reduction is good at early stages but most people tend to stray off track due to the high restrictions.

The common problem that people who follow low carbohydrate diets face is the absence of pasta and bread. No more spaghetti, pizza or toast! Most meals that are quick and easy to prepare revolve around carbohydrates - burger buns, sandwiches, fries and pasta. Beer, including other forms of alcohol is high in carbohydrate content. Generally, alcohol is restricted in all diet plans, but low carbohydrate diets emphasize on this point particularly, as they are high in calorie and low in nutrition.

There are still several foods that may be relished even when one is on a low carbohydrate diet. Meat lovers can grab the chance to consume chicken, beef and other poultry products. The popularity and effect of these diets are indicated by how long they remain on the list of bestsellers. But in the end, it depends entirely on what suits you. However, low carbohydrate diet plans seem to work for most people.

Overnight Weight Loss

With the rapid pace in which the world is advancing, it has become almost impossible to eat healthy and balanced food all the time. People have got more used to eat foods from fast-food haunts and other places thereby resulting in excessive consumption of low fiber food and refined sugar by way of different varieties of processed and tinned food and sodas and other unhealthy beverages. This has resulted in a large amount of the population around the world to be classified as obese or overweight.

There are many other factors which may result in obesity such as overeating, genetics and slow down of metabolism as a person grows older. The rate of weight loss is proportionate to the amount of weight gained.

Speedy weight loss is not considered sensible as it would make the skin of the person sag thereby making him adopt for a surgery to make the skin look better. Weight loss also depends on the health, weight, gender, age, calorie intake, stress level, routine and lifestyle.

All overweight people are not unhealthy but are considered to be unfashionable. One important and significant fact to be noted is that there is no instantaneous or miraculous weight loss solution available.

According to health experts and nutritionists adequate exercise with a balanced diet would be of great help in losing a few pounds every week. A proper workout schedule coupled with a low calorie diet program would help in achieving favorable results.

For this purpose, the individual should opt for a suitable diet plan designed by a health professional or a dietician according to the routine and lifestyle of the individual. Such plans have to be formulated in such a way that it does not comprise of purchase any costly fitness equipment or any kind of diet supplement.

A combination of weight training and cardiovascular workout exercise program would be very effective and helpful. This would help in increasing muscle to fat ratio on one hand and at the same time help in burning the extra fat thus inducing weight loss and an increase in the metabolism rate.

A balanced diet plan must consist of food items from all the varieties of food groups. This consists of two parts: 1. carbohydrates 2. Fats
The food consumed by an individual must comprise of fiber, minerals and vitamins in the right proportions. A lot of this can be taken by way of cereals, oats and potatoes. However, the best sources for this are fruits and vegetables as they contain photochemical, micronutrients and enzymes which are important for a balanced diet.

The second part comprises of fats which can come from poly saturated or mono saturated food stuff rather than that derived from animals. Proper care must be taken to consume fats in the correct quantity so that unwanted calories are not added.

Every diet plan is made keeping in mind lesser number of calories to be consumed by the individual. This refers to eating smart rather than starving or eating less by choosing the right food stuff in the right quantity. This helps in losing weight without eating less.

The individual should keep visiting the dietician or health professional throughout the diet period to see the improvement and keep track of the results achieved. This helps in making changes in the diet if necessary. However, by the end of it, it is in the hands of the individual to stick to diet plan strictly.

<u>Nine Facts About Fiber</u>

Looking for a diet that is high on octane, then you will happy to know that fiber is exactly the thing you need. People do not take this nutrient seriously even though research shows that it is powerful.

Here are nine important facts about fiber that will help you to fuel your health.

1. Fiber is a natural fighter of diseases. Diet that is rich in fiber helps in the prevention of colon cancer and diseases of the heart. Fiber also helps in the elimination of cholesterol by the action of binding it to the digestive tract. Fiber also helps in stopping constipation.

2. Fiber also helps in cooling of the body when it is over-heated. High fiber foods usually take longer to chew, thereby longer to digest and hence make you feel satisfied for a longer period of time.

3. The content of fiber in popular foods is very less. If you are used to depending on popular food then it is time to start increasing your fiber content.

4. Grains have the most content of fiber. The best sources of fiber are concentrated grain products and whole grains.

5. It is essential for kids to have fiber. Children older than two years should necessarily include fiber in their diet as they are the most receptive towards fiber in fruits, fortified breakfast cereals and vegetables.

6. More the intake of fiber more is the intake of water. For fiber to move through the digestive tracts a lot of water is needed. When a diet rich in fiber is consumed a minimum of eight glasses per day are required per day.

7. The health benefits of fiber are not lost during cooking. While cooking fruits and vegetables there is no need to worry about losing the fiber content. The fiber found in these fruits and vegetables isn't only in the skin.

8. Fiber must not be taken beyond a certain limit. A person must take more than 50 gms per day as this may lead to diarrhea and bloating and also interferes with the absorption of other minerals.

9. It is not hard to get the required amount of fiber content in your diet, even though the mis-conception is that, it is hard to get enough fiber into the diet. To get the right amount all you need to do is to eat the right kind of foods.

When you are determined to achieve a healthy lifestyle, eating fiber is something you do not want to miss as it serves more than one different purposes, most of which have been covered above

Atkins Induction Rules

The initial stage of any type of diet is the crucial factor which decides the effectiveness of the diet. So is the case with the Atkins diet. Along with the food items that can be consumed during the duration of the diet, there are certain golden rules which need to be followed during the diet period.

In the initial stages of dieting, it is recommended to people to consume three meals per day of regular size or five to six smaller meals is acceptable. If you tend to feel hungry very frequently, you can break your large meals into smaller segments. A vegetable and proteins diet would help in staying away from the craving to consume carbohydrates. Staying awake for a period more than six hours without a meal and skipping meals is not advisable at all.

There need not be any restriction on proteins and fats and you can freely choose to have a variety in the list of foods that are accepted. As the Atkins diet plan is not a diet restricting calories, you can go for as much as fats and proteins as you prefer. Only the level of carbohydrates in grams matters. It is necessary to calculate the amount of carbohydrates consumed in grams by way of cheese, beverages with splenda and vegetables. At least 12-15 grams of the carbohydrates intake which is allowed must be from vegetables. Vegetables play a major role when it comes to diet.

Whole fruits, pasta, grains, bread and vegetables with starch such as squash and cauliflower have to be avoided. Such food stuff will be introduced gradually with the passage of the diet. Beans have to be avoided as they contain carbohydrates along with proteins. If an urge to eat grain products is prevalent, low carbohydrate-high fiber food must be preferred. One thing to be noted here is that, this will slow down the process of weight loss.

During the introduction stage, it is completely out of question to have anything which is not in the list of acceptable foods. This is because; there is a great probability of it spoiling the whole diet plan.

The quantity of foods accepted should be adjusted as per the needs of individual appetite. As the craving for sugar and carbohydrates decreases, hunger pangs would gradually decrease. After this is achieved, only the satisfying amount of food must be consumed.

Special care must be taken to go through the labels of packaged food items even if it is specified that it is carbohydrate-free. This is because many products may contain hidden carbohydrates. If the percentage of fat is lesser than .5 percent, it can be rounded off as zero, by the manufacturer as the law does not prohibit it. The ingredients of the product may help in determining the presence of carbohydrates, if any. While having meat and salads care must be taken to ensure that carbohydrates are not consumed unknowingly by means of gravies and salad dressings. For this purpose, salads can be had with vinegar or olive oil dressing and meat can be had without gravy.

The next thing to be followed is to drink at least 8-ounces of water a day other than any other drink that you consume. This will help in avoiding constipation and would help in keeping the body hydrated. In the same way, the by-products of burnt fat can be flushed out of the body.

These are the golden rules which ought to be followed while starting off with the Atkins diet so that the desired results are achieved in the longer run.

<u>Overcoming Plateaus On The Atkins Diet</u>

It is common to experience plateaus and stalls during Atkins' diets. It occurs time and again, but, it is important to check whether you have actually come to the plateau point.

When you continue for a prolonged period of time, without losing any weight, it is called a plateau. It is essential to make a note of your weight and your measurements, before starting a diet plan. In the first couple of weeks, you may feel that you have not lost any weight but a quick glance at your measurements may lift your spirits.

The theory behind Atkins Diet is adding muscle to the body, by removing fat. This may result in slight weight gain because you are developing dense muscle to replace fat. You may end up adding a few pounds on the scale but you will shed those extra inches. You may obtain a leaner body but weigh just the same.

Take measurements of you waist, chest, calves, thighs, upper arms and hips before starting the diet program, because it is possible to lose weight in any of these areas and having comprehensive information is vital. It is not abnormal to go through times when your body needs to adjust. You must remember that as you are changing your body's composition, the process may be a little time consuming. Keep a weekly check on your measurements and your weight, so that you can keep track of your progress.

There are 3 to 4 week periods when you may experience plateaus in weight reduction, but you still continue to lose inches, or even vice versa. Checking both methods is an effective way to monitor your progress. These plateaus are no reason to give up on the diet. Such stall periods are common in weight loss programs.

Stalls are more frequent when you are just a couple of pounds away from your goal. You would have developed plenty of muscle by adopting this high protein and low carbohydrate plan. As your body's muscle-to-fat percentage has increased greatly, your body may resist anymore fat loss. At this point, you must reconsider your goal weight. Understand what your body is telling you and focus on maintaining your lost weight instead of trying to shed more and more weight.

On the path to weight loss, there are several other reasons behind the occurrence of stalls. If you have made no progress in four weeks and are not moving towards your goal weight, start looking at different methods to move out of the rut. Ensure that your level of carbohydrate in the body is in check. Intake of excess carbohydrate may cause plateaus in your weight loss. Watch out for hidden carbohydrate in dressing, sauces and packaged food.

Always have enough water. If your body gets dehydrated, it tends to retain water and will simulate a plateau. Water aids in flushing ketones and creating space for new ketones that help in burning fat.

Eating very less amount of food may also cause weight loss plateaus. Always have smaller meals at frequent intervals. You are following a low carbohydrate diet and not a low calorie diet. Always add enough protein to you meals. Do not go without food for more than five hours at a stretch. Do not keep check of your calorie intake because if your body does not get enough calories, it will switch to starvation mode and the fat cells get retained.

Increasing your fitness routine also helps in overcoming plateaus. Since your muscles are now accustomed to vigorous workouts, it is necessary to steadily intensify your workouts in order to challenge your body. Adding new routines or increasing weights during resistance training are good options.

One of these methods will help you get back on track with your weight loss program. These occasional plateaus and stalls are normal and do not last for long.

Ph Miracle Diet Basics

The latest path breaking invention to strike the world of nutrition and dieting is the pH Miracle Diet. Experts have noted that popular dieting plans seem to vary from time to time. For instance, the 90s marked lo-fat diets, and the last decade has focused on low-carbohydrate diets like Protein Power, South Beach diet, Sugar busters and Atkins. People begin to get frustrated with each new diet and start looking for newer options. The pH miracle has stolen the spotlight currently.

This diet appeals to most people as it completely different from the usual high- protein, low carbohydrate diets that have ruled the last couple of years. The pH diet, also known as the Young Diet, named after its founder Dr. Robert Young, or the alkaline diet, has a unique approach towards the supply of nutrition. Many medical experts, nutritionists and doctors find this diet program as an extremely balanced approach to achieve nutrition that considers the true requirements of the body.

Normally, our bodies have a slightly alkaline pH value. The principle is that as our body functions best at alkaline pH; our diet must be comprised of alkaline foods. The normal diet of an average American contains several acidic foods, including sugar caffeine, animal protein and packaged food. These acidic products disturb the pH level of the human body and thereby cause a myriad of problems. The principles of this diet claim that acidic foods hinder the benefits of alkaline minerals, including potassium, calcium, sodium and magnesium, which make people vulnerable to chronic conditions.

The real essence of the pH diet
Nutrition and health experts have realized that the food which a person consumes as part of his diet has a distinct effect on his overall health pattern. Though the medical community has given special importance to a balanced, nutritional diet which includes fresh fruits and vegetables, dairy and meat items, the pH diet is a step ahead. It clearly indicates that acidic foods deprive the body of its essential minerals. People, who adopt the pH miracle diet, have learnt to avoid intake of food that causes disastrous effects to health.

Most foods that we commonly consume are strictly forbidden in the pH diet. The most surprising of these restrictions is the removal of wheat products. Though the FDA suggests consumption of whole wheat products, the pH diet claims that grains like millet, wheat, rice and oats are harmfully acidic. Alkaline grains such as quinoa, spelt and buckwheat are favored due to their alkalizing benefits.

Usually, dairy and meat products are banned from the pH miracle Diet. For your protein source, goat milk is allowed. Protein is also available in tofu, nuts, seeds and beans. Almost all vegetables, except mushroom, have a high alkalizing effect. Intake of fruits is limited to grapefruit, lime, lemon and coconuts.

People who have adopted the pH miracle diet claim that there had been tremendous effect on their health well within the first couple of weeks. It is advisable to lower the consumption of pre-processed foods, and increase the intake of vegetables, irrespective of what the diet specifies for the person. As a matter of fact, this has become the point of major criticism of the pH diet. Opponents claim that those who are already consuming fresh food and plenty of water will find no effect from this diet. They ignore the pH balance theory.

Another significant point to be noticed is that there is no scientific proof of the theories involved in pH miracle diet. Several conventional doctors find no benefits arising from this diet. But the principles of this diet are based completely on Chinese medicine, which has been in practice for centuries. These proponents are currently being studied at the John Hopkins' University and by the United Nations. Critics may have to amend their attitude towards the basis of the diet.

Is The Ph Miracle Diet Right For You

The latest groundbreaking new invention to enter the field of nutrition and dietics is the pH Miracle Diet. This new method claims to help in restoration of your natural health balance and also rid you of innumerable other conditions, including obesity. Though most people are looking at efficient ways to lose a couple of pounds, this diet claims to aid dealing with muscle pain, indigestion and fatigue, along with several other problems.

If you've experimented low carbohydrate diets and found the excess protein levels staggering, then pH miracle diet program may be the answer to your woes. This program is primarily based on intake of alkaline foods, which benefit your body and health in more ways than one. As humans generally tend to have a mildly alkaline pH, consuming alkaline foods will help in maintaining the ph balance of the body. Many people eat acidic foods like meat, dairy and wheat products. The pH diet comprises of fruits, veggies, grains and vegetarian sources of protein.

The pH diet program is the brain child of Dr. Robert Young, who clearly indicates in his dieting book that excess acidity is the main cause behind most health related problems. Young says that nasal congestion, chronic fatigue, dry hair, weak nails, frequent cold infections, dry skin, stress, anxiety, muscle pain, headaches, arthritis, leg cramps and hives, among other disorders, are signs of high acid content in the body.

Your acidic diet can be held responsible if you have experienced any of these symptoms for a prolonged period of time. Keep a watch over the amount of acidic foods that you consume, including dairy products and animal protein. If these conditions have been a source of distraction and annoyance to your healthy lifestyle, then pH miracle is probably your best solution.

For people who have had little success with low carbohydrate diets, pH miracle diet program is an extremely relieving option. These alkaline foods are not as harsh as protein rich substances in low carbohydrate diets, and do not damage the digestive system. It possesses a healthier balance of protein-carbohydrate content. The proteins consumed in pH miracle program are carefully selected based on their acid level. It mainly consists of tofu, nuts and beans.

This diet program is also highly recommended for people who prefer to thrive on vegetarian food. If sacrificing meat products for a day has made you feel good, this pH diet is probably just the thing for you. There is absolutely no meat involved, and the sole dairy product allowed is goat's milk. Tofu, the major constituent of a vegetarian diet plays an essential role in the pH miracle diet.

If your diet is composed mainly of pre processed foods and negligible amounts of vegetables, this is the right option for you. Manufactured foods will not supply your body with the necessary nutrients. This may result in several health problems including malnutrition in spite of eating your fill. This Miracle pH diet focuses on fresh fruits and vegetables which will provide the required amount of vitamins and mineral to your diet. Adding a reasonable amount of alkaline meals to your diet program can bring drastic change to you health.

This pH miracle diet is found to be suitable for most kinds of persons. If you belong to any of the above mentioned categories, you simply must give this eating program a try.

pH Miracle Diet - Criticism

Whenever something gets famous, it gets criticized by some sources. The newly famous pH miracle diet isn't any different. The program has got followers, and it has also got a lot of criticism from a lot of people.

The first criticism about the diet is the fact that it asks people to be vegans and vegetarians. Critics claim that the diet, especially with its deletion of dairy products (vegetarian source of protein), is very low in protein content. However, this comes from the misconception that we need a large amount of proteins. Going by popularity of the low carbohydrate diet (that is just high in protein diets) has aggravated this conception in the heads of people. Sadly health has become equal to eating dairy and red meat.

Anyway, there are lots of sources of healthy proteins which don't contain the bad acidic effects of dairy products or red meat. In reality, many people take too much of protein and not too less. Generally women need around 45 grams per day, and a man needs around 55 grams. One cup of tofu (that is acceptable on pH diet) has around 20 gm of proteins. And beans have around 8 grams every half a cup. So in reality its easy to gain enough of protein from a vegetarian diet.

One more criticism about this issue is about calcium. Most people tend to equate drinking milk and getting stronger bones. But , American women take average two pounds of milk every day and still about 30 million women get osteoporosis. If taking milk made bones stronger, then only the opposite will be true. From a study done by Cornell nutritionist named Amy Joy Lanou who proved that there is no link between dairy substances and healthy bones in young adults and children. There are many sources of calcium in alkalizing food products which will enhance protection to osteoporosis.

Most critics also say that the importance on fresh foods and vegetables is the actual cause behind the victory that many get from diets. pH miracle diet recommends to eat around 70 percent of vegetables and some needed fruits. In this rate, no matter if you are consuming alkalizing food , anybody will see an enhancement in their health. Most critics disregard the need for the pH balance miracle diet.

But however, there are many people who experience good results after getting rid of wheat, which is an acidic food. Its not a product that one generally links with bad health, however, removing wheat has proved to be a godsend to loads of people who suffer the effects of an over-acidified meal. The quantity of alkalizing vegetables present in diet will surely do anyone good, no matter if they take the other parts of the diet seriously. By following eating of alkaline products, you would be enhancing the health irrespective of strictness of diet.

But this causes another famous criticism in the book. Most people say that pH miracle diet is way too strict for daily following. The reduction of foods like milk, animal protein and wheat seems too much for some. They can't imagine making it through a full day without consuming these food groups. Idea of restricting to a diet containing plant based food only seems too strict. However, most people who utilize pH miracle diet are seeing good results without having to be 100% rigid about the rules.

Like most other diets, pH miracle diet recommends steps to a better health. Emphasis here is on the steps. It's not reasonable to ask anyone for a total 180-degree change about his or her meal habits. Using a slower method for changing the diet will give longer and successful end results. If any diet is done word by word, it's very difficult at the start because mostly people are used to eating in a certain pattern. But with time and some practice , anyone can get better health through more of a H balanced diet.

Like with many other diets, the pH miracle diet outlines steps toward better health. The emphasis here is on steps. It is unreasonable to expect anyone to do a complete 180-degree change in his or her eating habits overnight. Taking a slower approach to changing your diet will create longer and more successful results. If the diet is followed word for word, it is difficult at first because people are so used to eating a certain way. With time and practice though, you can move toward better health and a more pH balanced diet.

Atkins Pre Maintenance Phase

The pre maintenance stage comes after the orientation and OWL stages of the diet plan. This stage is the stepping stone to a balanced and healthy living for all the years to time. This should be begun when you are within five to ten pounds nearer to the target you have set. This would slow down the weight loss process but you will learn techniques which would help you in achieving better results in the long-run.

In the OWL stage, you would slowly start introducing little grams of carbohydrates to your diet which would be gradually increased by 5 grams each week. When the pre-maintenance week starts, this increment would be increased to 10 grams every week. Carbohydrate grams are added till the time you lose weight however slow it may be. Generally, it is common to lose less than one pound every week in the pre-maintenance phase.

This state should be carried on till you reach your target weight and successfully maintain it at least for a month, as per the Atkins diet plan book. The duration of this process ranges from one to three months. The target to be achieved is termed as the stage of "carbohydrate equilibrium" and is the state when your carbohydrate intake is perfect and would help in maintaining the desired weight in the longer run.

A wide range of food items can be had during this period. New food stuff can be introduced gradually and intake of carbohydrates has to be increased side by side at a properly calculated rate. Increasing the intake of carbohydrates by ten grams every week is considered ideal. This would help in maintaining the ideal weight.

Before adding a new item into the diet, it is necessary to check up the carbohydrate counter book or a website. Some food items which contain ten gram carbohydrates are half an apple, quarter cup of potatoes, one-third cup of legumes, and half a cup of plain oatmeal. Such foods are to be included on a day to day basis, and then have to be increased with the passing weeks.

Pre-maintenance cannot be termed as a complete process. It takes a subtle balance of exercise and carbohydrate counting to decelerate the weight loss and still move forward. Enough care should be taken to keep an eye on the carbohydrate intake so that it does not result in weight gain in any way. There is a thin line which separates gaining, losing and maintaining weight. Pre-maintenance is the period when you are looking for this fine line.

If weight loss cannot be stalled while adding on carbohydrates, it implies a great metabolic resistance. In such a case exercises can prove beneficial when increased.

Another method which can be followed is treating oneself a couple of times a week by saving carbohydrate grams of some days. This can be done by consuming beer or white wine or by having a portion of sweet potatoes or a fruit piece. The other way is to calculate the carbohydrate intake per week and divide it in such a way that you consume a little less on a few days while you can have a blast on the other days using the quantity of carbohydrates that was saved. However, care should be taken to not let the carbohydrate craving increase again.

The pre maintenance stage is a sure shot way for long term results if followed properly. It would help in maintaining the weight as well as have a balance over the carbohydrate intake.

<u>Teen Dieting</u>

21st century has seen the largest number of obese teenagers and children all around the world since the start of time. The fast food and coffee pub culture has made them lethargic and inactive. Many parents prefer to keep their children at home for safety reasons which makes them even more inactive and lazy and in turn results in them becoming couch potatoes who can spend hours together in front of the idiot box or the computer. These things, rather than making them better, wrecks havoc on their health.

Teenagers of today are invariably spending most of their time over the phone or in front of computers and televisions. This has made them lazy, inactive unhealthy and unfit. It has also left a huge impression on the diet, exercise and nutrition patterns that they follow.

For this purpose, many games have been introduced in the markets which have been aimed at giving some sort of exercise to the teenagers within the four walls. Games such as the brand new Nintendo wii system of gaming and the Dance party Revolution of Play station 2 have created an impact in the market in this regard. They are a fun way to stay in shape in the way teenagers prefer it. Such games provide an opportunity for them to get involved with it totally rather than the video games which used to be played in a static environment. This encourages active participation of the youngsters and is therefore equally popular among adults as a great stress buster and workout session.

"All work and no play make Jack a dull boy". This old saying holds absolutely well. In this rapidly growing and improving world, children and teenagers need to be encouraged to get active and get out. Adolescents learn by instances and whether they accept it or not, they thoroughly enjoy doing activities along with family members. Such activities must thus be encouraged. Family outings must be planned including activities like mountain climbing, wall climbing, biking, hiking, and boating and so on. You can also plan camps during weekends or learn any new activity or sport together. Any activity that is taken up by the teenager must be encouraged so that he/she does not lose interest in it and is actively involved in it.

You can also encourage your teenage daughter or son to join a club for any sport they like. They can play games which they already know or can join some new sport about which they are interested and keen to know. A family match of soccer or volleyball or softball is also a great way of inducing physical activity as well as fun and gives an opportunity for everyone in the family to get some sort of physical exercise.

Gardening is another great way to have fun as well as to burn a few calories. Try to identify activities which your teen kid enjoys and try to encourage them in it. Work with them together and keep boosting them for their work which would keep them happy as well as engaged in the activity thereby keeping them active. It is a great way to unwind rather than sitting in front of the television or the computer which would make them consume more calories by way of unhealthy snacking.

They must also be encouraged to consume more nutritious food and to exclude carbonated beverages, energy drinks and artificial fruit juices and other oily and starchy snack items. Include more of fresh fruits and vegetables in their diet and make sure they drink lots of water. Make them participate in activities such as cooking and serving and clearing tables. This would help them in understanding what is healthy and what is not and thus help in inculcating better eating habits in them.

The Dieting Mind Set

Dieting is a process which involves a great deal of will power. This is because a number of restrictions exist during the duration of the plan. This is the reason why many people do not succeed when it is concerned with their diet plans. This has made many people dread the idea of dieting as they always have the dumb intuition that they would not be able to follow the routine resulting in many diet plans to fail even before they are started.

Many people fail to understand that healthy dieting does not refer to starving. This is one major reason for many people to not take up dieting as they think they will have to completely stay away from food which they love. They are not making it clear to themselves that they can moderately eat food stuff which they like and cannot completely give up. This is why many people are totally against dieting as they confuse the term with starving themselves.

People should know that if a diet plan they adopt has to be successful, then they have to change their view on the food they prefer eating and must compromise with their personal likes for a certain period of time. Again, one more thing which people do not seem to understand is that food is not our enemy but our inability to correctly divide and consume it, is. Very often, most of the population ends up eating the wrong foods more than the correct foods which ought to be consumed. This is the epicenter of the problem.

Five portions of veggies and three of fruits is the right amount of food that we must consume everyday for getting the right quantity of nutrients necessary. If this is not fulfilled, we tend to feel deprived and suffer hunger pangs. If we correctly consume the above mentioned servings of fruits and vegetables, we are unlikely to have frequent hunger pangs. This implies we can enjoy the food we love in moderations as it has to be.

The size per serving is another major problem o deal. We are so used to eat the extra large pack of fries and the large cup of colas and other beverages that we fail to understand what the correct serving size is. All such temptations must be avoided and only what is needed must be consumed.

We must make it a point to always remember that dieting is not starving and hence must feel good about the whole process and motivate ourselves to take it up. All the positive aspects of dieting and weight loss must be kept in mind always rather than feeling low about the excess weight you are carrying with you now. A positive outlook of the whole thing is to be adopted and you must keep motivating yourself even if the process of losing weight is taking longer than expected. Keep telling it to yourself that you would be getting your youthful body back.

However, dieting does not mean you should completely stop enjoying things which you liked. You can treat yourself to some goodies once in a while in moderation. After this, for burning the extra calories that you have consumed choose an activity which you cherish and enjoy. This way, you get double the benefit. The exercises you have taken up must be something which you look forward to and enjoy. This would help in achieving better results.

To be a successful 'dieter', you need to be confident and have a positive approach towards the whole dieting program. If you cannot keep yourself away in case of indulging, then it is better to avoid indulging however tough it may be. Nonetheless, if you are happy and feel good about the whole concept of dieting and exercise and keeping fit, then having little treats in moderation once in a while is a great option.

The Greatest Dieting Mistakes

As far as dieting is considered mistakes are made almost on a daily basis, some of these mistakes are real and profound, some go with the territory, but there are few mistakes that have a more lasting implication than others. The only way to avoid these mistakes is by learning about them and avoiding them during the course of your weight loss regime.

The biggest mistake made by dieters is adopting the strategy of all or nothing. These dieters remove anything from the pantry that they consider will give room for the slightest of temptations. After doing this the dieters start on a strict dietary regime that is not only difficult but nearly impossible to continue, believing that they lose every thing the moment they stray away from their military like diet regime.

The above method may work for a few people but it will lead to un-wanted anger, frustration and sometimes even failure. The most important thing in relation to the dieting regime is the goal. What is the goal for dieting? The answer is shedding those extra pounds. There is more than one way of achieving your target without half starving to death or pushing yourself to the brink.

Another big mistake in relation to dieting is the selection of diet plan. Some people make the mistake of selecting a plan that involves eating the same food everyday. Human beings enjoy change and will get frustrated with routine, therefore it is necessary to change our pattern once in a while. You can do this by choosing a diet regime that allows for a wider variety of food rather than one which limits the number of choices.

Some of the other common mistakes are depriving yourself of all the food we enjoy. Moderation is the key word here. Have a diet that is rich in fruits & vegetables but also do not forgot to indulge yourself once in a while to keep yourself going and sane. The important thing here is not to forget enjoying food while dieting, if you enjoy eating chocolates then why would you want to deprive yourself of eating them. There is nothing sinful or wrong about eating the food you like, but the problem is that most people enjoy the wrong sort of food.

Never make the commonly made mistake of not setting any goals. While setting goals it is important to remember that one should never set goals that are almost impossible to achieve, on the other hands you must not follow a regime in which practically no goals are achieved. The key here is setting goals that are achievable, these have the most likelihood of attaining success. Making these goals public and requesting support isn't a bad idea either. This is the prime reason for the stupendous success that has been achieved by weight watchers program.

It is also important during the course of a dietary regime never to get frustrated and give up. Set backs are common and are faced by almost all people, even the ones who have achieved stunning dieting regime success have met with failure en route. The end result is that you end up getting an healthier body and something worth fighting for. Sometimes your goals may go off track but it always possible to set new goals and start afresh. Somewhere down the road you may have a couple of bad day or sometimes a bad week even in relation to your dieting regime. This should not be a deterrent to your plans, instead you must overcome them in order to see a healthier you.

Learn from the mistakes you make, overcome them and move on fast. Failures should teach you as much as success does. Once you learn from these failures you are well on track to achieving an healthier persona. Irrespective of the amount of weight you plan to lose you must dedicate yourself to the task of losing weight. Also remember a healthy person is one who has good heating habits and not one who tries to starve himself. Select a moderate approach and you are well on the road to success.

Vegetarianism And The PH Miracle Diet

The miracle diet is a regime which helps to restore balance in our body by consuming alkaline foods. The cells of the body are naturally alkaline and you can enhance your body's natural function by consuming alkaline foods. Adding on to this consumption, Dr.Robert Young, who created the diet, recommends omitting acidifying items like wheat, dairy and meat. Becoming vegetarians is a must for those who want improved health, according to Dr. Young. He accepts that the change to vegetarianism requires a lot of mental control and strength.

The diet which is most standard in America is not devoid of alkalizing food and is not vegetarian. Animal proteins are inevitable in the diet of people. Despite, there is no compulsion to consume animal protein. It could be well compensated by the protein rich sources available in the vegetarian group.

A belief prevails in our society that the physical well-being and health of an individual is encouraged by proteins. Especially men, are demanded to consume huge quantities of meat to have vitality and strength. This figment has however prevailed for a long time. As early as the 20th century, scientists believed that consumption of meat equaled strength, prominently in the field of sport. This myth has essentially been the driving force behind meat eating in the last century.

In reality, the need for protein by a person's body is less than assumed by most people. The sources of vegetarian proteins are plenty and are acceptable on the miracle pH diet. There are plenty of sources from which an individual can choose.

But why is animal protein forbidden by this program? Dairy, meats and eggs which are sources of animal protein, have acidifying significance on our body. This tends to prevail on consumption of non-organic meat.

Consumption of processed meat can lead to exposure of hormones, chemicals and drugs being given to animals before they are killed. Risks of the hormones prevail as there are no definite studies about them. Our consumption of antibiotics will increase as the animals are periodically fed with them. this increased consumption will lead to reduction of helpful bacteria in our body. This leads to accumulation of metabolic acid in our system, leading to disastrous effects. The helpful bacteria which check the accumulation of metabolic acid in our system are killed by the antibiotics in the animals.

Good elements like minerals, vitamins and proteins can be obtained from vegetarian food without any dangers.20 grams of protein is contained in a cup of tofu, which is an alkalizing source. An average human requires only about 40 gm of protein per day. This can be easily satisfied without the consumption of meat.

Switching to vegetarianism is much of a mental battle than a physical battle. In fact, the absence of acidifying animal protein leads to efficient body. Consumption of meat is a routine and the advantages of consuming it is a figment. There is no need for meat physically. Omitting meat from our diet leads to opening our eyes to a huge variety of foods that convincingly replace meat.

When one follows the miracle diet, he/she will notice that Dr.Robert suggests an equity of 70 percent alkaline, and 30 percent acidic food. Hence, there is some extent for consuming items in the acidic group. Even though it would be tempting to consume proteins from animal sources, it is preferable to choose from the less acidic foods like oats, eggs, pastas and other products.

It is certainly the individual's choice to become a pure vegetarian. Reducing the quantity of animal protein will lead to improvements in your health eventually.

What Is In A Weight Loss Diet Pill?

Most programs for weight loss have really strict regimes and strenuous activities and for this reason a lot of people prefer to opt for some other alternative without having to go through the effort of exerting themselves too much.

So, it can easily be understood how diet pills with their promises of simply 'melting away' your cellulite and fat in a jiffy, appeals to most people and they are strongly tempted to resort to these pills.

When there is such an easy method of loosing weight, who would want to go through the effort of building biceps and abs through exercise and diet?

Today, 60% of Americans are said to be obese. It is no surprise then, how the manufacturers of these 'wonder' drugs target this population. In the US alone, these companies are earning millions of dollars.

There are many questions. Are the manufacturers' claims about their drug being able to help in weight loss true? How effecting are these drugs in actually making people lose weight? Suppose it is true, do these drugs help in the maintenance of the ideal weight and prevent future weight gain?

It is true that there exist diet pills that make people shed extra pounds. They contain many substances that have been scientifically and clinically proven to show results.

The diet pill functions by causing an increase in the body metabolism and thereby causing weight loss. Also these pills contain substances that can suppress a person's appetite.

But with the numerous diet pills in the market today, it is getting tougher to make a right decision about which pill to choose. People mostly lose patience and end up buying the wrong diet pill.

There are, actually, only five things to consider while choosing a diet pill that is effective as well as safe to consume. Below is a list that you might find helpful in choosing a diet pill that's appropriate and right.

1.   Metabolism boosting ability

Metabolism is your body's ability to burn fat. While looking for a diet pill, it is advisable to choose a pill that has ingredients that increase body metabolism.

You might want to choose a pill that has alpha lipoic acid, "L-Canitine' and green tea extracts because all these ingredients have been proven to be clinically effective in increasing weight loss by increasing metabolic rate.

2.   Appetite suppressants

Go for appetite suppressing diet pills. People often think that these pills will make them skip meals. The pill simply stops you from feeling hungry too often. Excess calorie intake is initiated when people take meals at odd hours and in between meals and this leads to obesity.

3.   The Calorie stopper

Obesity is caused when more than the recommended amounts of calorie are consumed in excess and hence it is important to choose diet pills that have substances that can curb calorie intake into the body.

These ingredients are called 'phaseolus vulgaris'. This creates an enzyme that can efficiently control excess calories from entering the body. The enzyme in question is called 'alpha amylase'.

4.   Metabolic enhancers

The best diet pills are those that have 'lipotropic' elements that are known to eliminate fat from the body. It functions somewhat similar to a sweeper that sweeps away the excess fat from the body.

Lipotropic elements are present in vitamin C, green tea extracts, alpha lipoic acid and chitosan.

5.   Water-retention breaker

Diet pills that contain diuretics are supposed to be very effective. During the weight loss program, it is these elements that avert water retention in the body.

All these factors are effective in weight loss and are clinically proven. But it is not enough to take diet pills to lose weight. Exercise is still very important. Hence with the correct diet pill and exercise you are definitely headed to a slimmer and healthier life.

Weight Reduction Drugs

It is shown in research that the percentage of healthy and fit people is reducing to the percentage of people who are unfit. The major cause of this fitness deficiency is caused due to the rise in obese people. More shockingly patient who suffer from obesity are not only from the adult sector, it includes children starting from an age of ten. The factor that causes such obesity issue varies from eating habits to genetics. What concerns the doctors is that, if children at an age of ten develop obesity it will become harder for that person to get rid of it in the later stage due to the slow down of metabolic rate.

Thankfully, due to the advancement in the medical science field it is possible to solve obesity issue in many ways. The patient has the choice ranging from surgery to changing eating habits, depending on the will of the patient. It is always favorable for the patient to use the fastest way out – weight loss drugs.

Started as early as 1950, drugs were prescribed for weight loss. These drugs work by increasing the level of serotonin making the brain believe that the stomach is full, effectively increasing the metabolic rate.

Soon after in 1990, side effects of these drugs were discovered, example heart valve disease. This led to the expulsion of the drugs. Since then newly developed drugs require the FDA approval, many of which are still in the waiting list. The way in which the drug works is simple, it changes the body with out need to change in diet or avoiding anything tempting to eat.

This industry has made large amount of profit from the consumer. The drugs are easily available either over-the –counter or simply prescribed by the doctor. However the side effects are still eminent. The patient can go through many unpleasant experiences such as diarrhea, vomiting even urinary problems, the most fatal being heart attack or a stroke. Overdose can even cause hallucinations or convulsions.

Depending on the habits of the patient, side effects vary. It is always worth to consult a doctor before any purchase of weight reduction drugs. These are just the physical side effects, research shows mental stability can also be affects, as the patient may go through mood swings, nightmares, depression and even severe irritation.

Clinical study shows that weight reduction drugs work efficiently with the help of a low calorie diet along with routine exercise. The diet must have food from all groups. Phytochemicals, micronutrient and enzymes from fruits and vegetable are essential. Other sources of food group such as the vitamins fiber and minerals are also important for the body to have a healthy diet and stay fit.

Exercising is also important, one could workout regularly at the nearby gym or just prefer to go for a long walk every morning. Doctor must be consulted to do the right amount and the right intensity of exercise everyday. The exercise must include cardiovascular (for the heart) and weight training (for the loss of weight). They help to reduce calories inside the body and reduce the percentage of fat in our body. By doing so, the amount of fat to muscle will reduce helping to increase the metabolism rate in our body and stay fit.

Weight Loss Plan

Generally excess fat holds you at risk of getting many health related problems, you have get weight loss plans in order to avoid these risks and also to prevent disease.

What is the long-term goal? What about short-term goals u need to set in order to get there? You will have a much better chance of reaching all the goals if you can just make sure these plans that you might utilize are reasonable and sensible.

Some of the guidelines given by experts for choosing the correct plan.

1. Try To Be realistic

Many people's long-term plans are very ambitious more than what is has to be.

Like for example, incase you weigh around 170 pounds and the plan is to reduce to 120, although you haven't weighed that much since 16 and now nearly 45, which isn't a proper goal.

The body mass index called in short BMI is a very good indicator to know if you have to shed some weight. The proper BMI variation range, according to certain international sources, is anywhere from 19 till 24.9. Incase your BMI is anywhere from 25 to 29.9, you should consider yourself overweight. All numbers above 30 range is the obesity range.

According to point of view, people need a sane weight loss plan which will correlate to the needed BMI according to your height, since this is the main factor that affects your BMI levels.

2. Set reasonable objectives

Trying a weight loss idea for just vanity's sake is mentally a little less helpful than to lose weight to enhance health.

A huge step forward has been made if you decide and undertake a proper weight loss plan which includes eating right and exercise to make you will feel much better and also to have energy to do positive things in life.

3.Try and Focus on doing it, not losing it

Instead of saying that you will lose at least a pound by end of this week, its better to say how much exercise you get done this week. That would surely make a sane plan.

Do keep in thought that the weight in a span of a week isn't totally under your control, only your behavior surely is.

4. Try and Build in bits

Ant short term plans for weight loss shouldn't be like "a pie-in-the-sky." Which means that if you haven't exercised in a while, the best plan for the week must be based on getting to know around three single mile routes to walk for the whole of the coming week.

5. Do Keep up the Motivation

A do or die attitude only ensures your failure. You must evaluate your efforts objectively and fairly. In case you don't complete some goals, let it go and move to next week. Perfect record is not needed.

Self encouragement must surely be part of the weight loss plans. If not, you might end up failing.

6. Always Use measurable attempts

Telling that you will be positive in the coming weeks or that you want to get serious this week are not goals which you can measure hence mustn't part of the weight loss plan.

That is yet another reason as to why you must include exercise on the plan and also focus on it. Anyone must be able to include 3 minutes of exercise time so as to be very successful in the plan. Bottom line is that, everyone must use plans which will remain just a plan. They must put it to action only by including goals which will encourage them to succeed.

Program Your Weight Loss In As Easy As A Week

The idea behind the program is for you to develop a uniform approach towards weight loss and also healthy endurance during exercising. This program's main aim is to reduce excesses in the body, like excess fat. But not healthy and slim muscle tissues and important body fluids which are very vital.

This program initially needs your dedication and focus , hence you have to be equipped in both the mind and the body. It is advised that first go to the doctor for a routine check-up prior to taking up weight loss programs.

It is needed that whenever starting on weight loss programs, you have to be sure enough to work towards the results. Many people tend to get impatient but long term results are guaranteed so long as one maintains to the plan devised for them taking into consideration their body condition and needs.

Try to stretch a lot. Prior to doing the exercises and also working out , some stretching is mandatory so that you avoid any kind of injury in the body.

It is not advised for anybody to try very hard. All things must be done in correct levels. Know the level of training and exercise that will suit you best. It has to be correct enough to be comfortable with but not too easy so that it won't be a challenge.

In the first week

First few days in the program needs long and steady walks for about twenty minutes. After walking, try to follow up stretching. This only takes little of the time in the first few days. Less than an hour or so you will have taken the first steps for any weight loss program which can work to your benefit.

In the second day, it's better to think about upper body workouts. This will maintain the strength to proceed with program for a whole week. And on third day, a bright jog or walk for about ten minutes is required. For new comers, lower body workouts must be taken up in evening time.

By the fourth day, good rest is required, along with a nice long stretch. The lag time must be used properly to correct out negatives thoughts in your mind. Start fifth day with a brisk ten minute of walk. Do exercises for the lower body in about four workout sessions, then take another walk for ten minutes, and do another round of four sessions workout for lower body.

The sixth day must be spent for less tough exercises like swimming. In order to get rid of boredom, do try anything new. The seventh day is the time to get the support of people you tend to care about. Do spend some time for them or bring them with you for the long walk. Also, do light upper body workouts after the walk so that you don't lose the warm up.

This is only the start. By the initial week if can to stick with the program, then you have a chance to boost the weight loss and also stay according to the plan till you reach the desired result. Do try not to be like some people who tend to give up easily because they can't see the end result in the time frame they hope - like this instant, today! Patience is the most important virtue. Think about how much your body will go through to get remove all the fat.

<u>Weight Watchers Dieting</u>

In the field of dieting and weight watching there are just a handful of organizations that have actually successfully achieved what they promise. These organizations seem to be on the roll and there is no question of stopping them. More significant are the people who join and manage to stick to it till the end. So why do some programs take the backseat while some steal the show?

Community

One chief reason behind the success of Weight Watchers is the sense of community, the bond that is forged between all the men and women who have a common goal-weight loss. It is encouraging as well as endearing to be with a set of people with whom you can share your experiences as well as theirs.

More often than not, people who are on diet or a program simply do not get enough support from their family and friends. The bonding that takes place in the meetings of the Weight Watchers is strong because it is of people who come from diverse walks of life and cultures but are still united under one common aim of losing weight and a leading healthier lives. And this bond is very dear to them because it is together that they laugh and cry. The kind of motivation and encouragement that this type of program stimulates is commendable to the highest degree.

Evolution

Though the typical manner in which to watch weight would be to actually attend the meetings, the community of Weight Watchers knows how to evolve with time. For those who are too busy or are just afraid to attend meetings, there are many alternatives available like online forums, support group sand message boards.

But the evolution has not stopped here. They have, in recent years, introduced a system of points which allows dieters to gauge how well they are performing or progressing through points instead of having to actually keep track of and account for every calorie. Counting every calorie is a hassle many dieters should not have to take time out of their busy schedules to sort out (especially while dining out).

The Weight Watchers online website is a great example of fast evolution in response to the ever changing requirements of men and women taking part in the program. They truly outdo themselves in terms of the information and insights offered.

Commitment to fitness

It is common knowledge among the Weight Watchers that dieting alone does not reap benefits. A diet in combination with an appropriate exercise gives much better and satisfying results. When it comes down to it, the most successful Weight Watchers are the ones who along with proper nutrition and attitude towards food, also stress on exercise as a vital component of the regime.

Weight Watchers is one among numerous other dieting and weight loss programs available in the market today. That they have carved a niche for themselves and are above many others in this particular field demands recognition. Despite the innumerable weight reduction programs being introduced every other month, Weight Watchers has consistently achieved laudable results for those who actually work at it. There are not many programs that can claim the same for themselves.

Considering all of the afore mentioned, along with the pre packaged food and extensive recipes offered by the Weight Watchers, coupled with their remarkable track record for success, there is no way you wouldn't want to at least check out what they have to offer you.

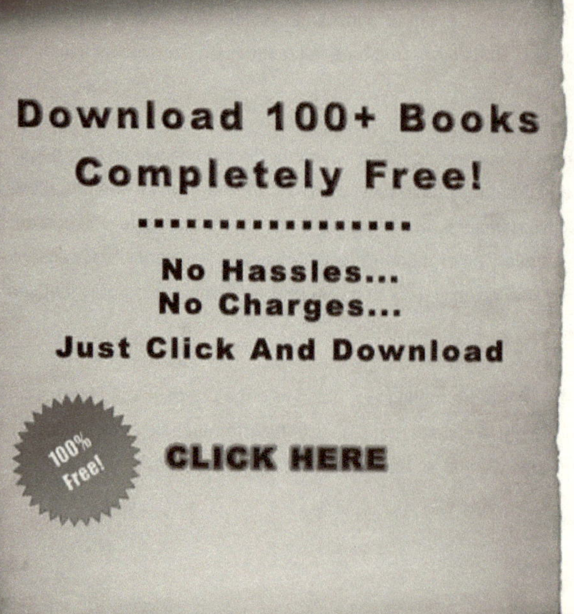
Download 100+ Books
Completely Free!
No Hassles...
No Charges...
Just Click And Download
100% Free!
CLICK HERE

This Product Is Brought To You By

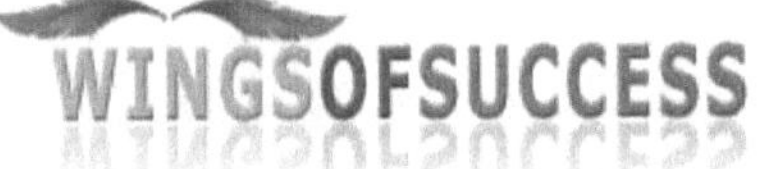